Clinical Record Book of Medical-Surgical Nursing

Clinical Record Book of Medical-Surgical Nursing

Second Edition

Himalayani Sharma
Master in Nursing (Delhi University)
Faculty, Ahilya Bai College of Nursing
New Delhi, India

Foreword
Amit Banerjee

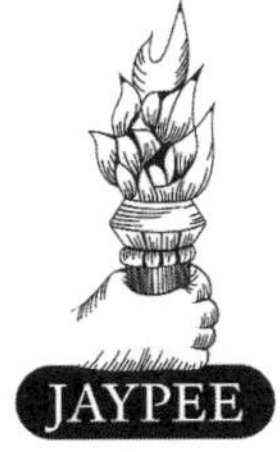

JAYPEE BROTHERS MEDICAL PUBLISHERS
The Health Sciences Publisher
New Delhi | London

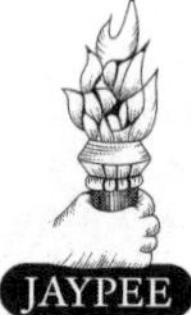

JAYPEE **Jaypee Brothers Medical Publishers (P) Ltd**

Headquarters
EMCA House
23/23-B, Ansari Road, Daryaganj
New Delhi 110 002, India
Landline: +91-11-23272143, +91-11-23272703
+91-11-23282021, +91-11-23245672
E-mail: jaypee@jaypeebrothers.com

Corporate Office
Jaypee Brothers Medical Publishers (P) Ltd.
4838/24, Ansari Road, Daryaganj
New Delhi 110 002, India
Phone: +91-11-43574357
Fax: +91-11-43574314
E-mail: jaypee@jaypeebrothers.com

Overseas Office
JP Medical Ltd.
83, Victoria Street, London
SW1H 0HW (UK)
Phone: +44-20 3170 8910
E-mail: info@jpmedpub.com

EU GPSR Authorised Representative
Logos Europe, 9 rue Nicolas Poussin
17000, La Rochelle, France
Phone: +33 (0) 6 67 93 73 78
E-mail: Contact@logoseurope.eu

Website: www.jaypeebrothers.com
Website: www.jaypeedigital.com

Clinical Record Book of Medical-Surgical Nursing

First Edition: **2011**
Second Edition: **2018**
Reprint: 2025, **2026**

ISBN: 978-93-5270-256-5

Printed at: Samrat Offset Pvt. Ltd.

Dedicated to

My Parents, Husband, Children and
Medical-Surgical Nursing Students

Foreword

The cornerstone of any accomplished technical skill in the field of medicine depends on the teaching-learning material available and the opportunity to have hands-on practice. Hands-on practice without a proper systematic guidance is like sailing on a rudderless boat. With the vast and relentless expansion of various avenues in the health care sector, it is not always possible to achieve transfer of skills through direct person-to-person interaction. It is in these situations that a well-crafted book can achieve wonders.

It gives me great pleasure to write an approbation of the present book on medical-surgical nursing. The book has been authored to create a step-by-step learning schedule for those who are seriously interested in mastering the art and science of nursing. Starting with the basic particulars of admission and discharge, going on to the rigorous demands of successfully and safely running an operation theater, the book has everything within its covers. It is a matter of great satisfaction that it covers even those areas which are mandatory under the NABH guidelines.

To me, it appears that the book will go a long way in fulfilling the much-needed requirement for a manual of this kind. For those who are interested in learning further about the historical aspects as well as recent progression in the field of medical-surgical nursing, there is a rich bibliography at the end. The success of this book will depend entirely on how an individual learner can use, utilize or exploit the pains that have gone behind the creation of this book.

Amit Banerjee
Vice Chancellor
Shiksha 'O' Anusandhan
Bhubneshwar, Odisha, India

Preface to the Second Edition

I am extremely delighted to present the second edition of *Clinical Record Book of Medical-Surgical Nursing*. The earlier edition was written as per the recommended course by Indian Nursing Council, but this edition was revised as per the syllabus of various universities across the country.

This edition has been enriched with entire text revision making the content more meaningful with a new additional chapter on gadgets. An attempt has also been made to supplement the text with pictures for better comprehension. The constructive feedback received from senior teachers have also been taken into consideration while revising the text.

I am very thankful to all the readers for their overwhelming response to the first edition and constructive suggestions for this edition. I sincerely hope that the readers would continue to communicate their valuable feedback in future also.

God Bless

Himalayani Sharma

Preface to the First Edition

It is our notion that a book is not a static document. Of course, a book-bound and printed reflects health care at a given moment of time. By making this *Clinical Record Book of Medical-Surgical Nursing,* I am able to provide the basic instructions and guidelines to deliver safe and effective nursing care to our patients.

Due to recent developments in health care services, the role of nurses has also become more elaborate. Despite these changes, it is important that the basics of nursing remain the foundation stone of practice. Nurses must be knowledgeable and professionally competent. They must be technically sound and personally caring.

It is this building of the new on the old that this *Clinical Record Book of Medical-Surgical Nursing* has been developed. It is the basic knowledge of nursing techniques and principles that will help the students to plan an effective strategy for their patients.

The primary aim of this book has been to help medical-surgical nursing students provide an excellent quality care to patients and their families. The contents of this text has been authored in a way that it devotes to most of the medical-surgical clients. The text in these chapters will guide the students to deliver a comprehensive care irrespective of the specific diagnosis or problem. A brief description of each chapter is given below:

Chapter 1 discusses the basic contents of health and disease, changing health status and the general pathophysiological changes that a body experiences as a result of an illness process.

Chapter 2 presents an overview of a client being admitted, transferred, discharged or going LAMA (leaving against medical advice) from a health agency.

Chapter 3 presents the five-step nursing process that serves as the organizing framework for all medical-surgical clients.

Chapter 4 discusses the health assessment. In this chapter, a detailed nursing health history and head-to-toe physical examination of medical-surgical patient is described.

Chapter 5 explains the diagnostic evaluation of these patients. A detailed description ranging from simple blood tests to advanced investigations is given in this chapter.

Chapter 6 looks at the concepts of perioperative nursing. This chapter gives details of nursing care required in the preoperative, intraoperative and postoperative phases of surgery.

Chapter 7 on pharmacological nursing, covers all the drug-related aspects of patient care. This chapter has a beautiful coverage of nursing components in drug administration.

Chapter 8 examines the complex nature of operation theater nursing. Section I in this chapter discusses the architectural, engineering and nursing components while Section II is all about the variety of operation theater instruments used in surgical procedures.

Chapter 9 presents the nursing case study and/or case presentation. This chapter follows the case study through the steps of nursing process, helping the students learn how to apply the process along with critical thinking, to the care of client.

Assignments in medical-surgical nursing form the backbone of clinical experience. Practical assignments on nursing care plans (15), nursing case studies (15), pharmacological nursing, operation theater nursing, observation reports (15) and a procedure record and simple and advanced medical-surgical procedures have been amalgamated sequentially to enrich the learning experience of our students.

Towards the end, I see this book as a 'work in progress' in guideline that would help all the medical-surgical students to proceed progressively in the care of their patients.

Further editions will definitely continue to improve, and I appreciate your comments, correction and doubts to guide my ongoing work. I can improve only with your input. I also strongly believe that students and teachers must work collaboratively to bring the book to life.

Himalayani Sharma

Acknowledgments

It requires great determination, interest and hard work to write a book. To achieve this task, encouragement, support, cooperation and blessings of many are essential.

This book is a result of many years of learning. I am deeply indebted to my teachers at Ahilya Bai College of Nursing and Rajkumari Amrit Kaur College of Nursing, New Delhi whose unique teachings and guidance helped me to develop an in-depth knowledge of the subject that has guided me in designing and preparing the manuscript of this record book.

I am grateful to my colleagues, faculty and students of various schools and colleges of nursing who expressed the need to have a comprehensive, standardized and practical-oriented record book of medical-surgical nursing. For this, I am particularly thankful to my students of ABCON.

I express my sincere thanks to Dr (Ms) Saroj Kumar, Vice Principal, ABCON for all the support she provided while writing this project.

I wish to acknowledge with gratitude Dr Amit Banerjee, Principal, ABCON, Director–Professor, Cardiothoracic Surgery, GB Pant Hospital and Medical Superintendent, Lok Nayak Hospital for the support and encouragement he provided while writing this manuscript. I am also grateful to him for writing foreword to this book and permitting me for the lavish photoshoot of surgical instruments in the OT block of the hospital. Very humbly I also acknowledge the efforts and cooperation of theater nurses during my visits.

I would like to extend my appreciation to M/s Jaypee Brothers Medical Publishers (P) Ltd, New Delhi, for having faith in me and turning my vision into reality. I am especially grateful to Mr Subrata Adhikary, Commissioning Editor and Ms Ruby Sharma, Project Manager who made the task of writing very simple by extending all the support as and when needed.

I humbly thank the staff of National Medical Library and my college librarian, Ms Sweena Gambhir for providing me with all the literature needed to furnish information in various chapters.

It was Mr Bharat Bhushan Vohra, who undertook the typing work of this manuscript in a very professional way. I warmly acknowledge his contribution.

An expression of sincere, deep and never-ending warm thanks to my parents, Mr Chunilal and Ms Prem, for their encouragement, and never-faltering support. I warmly express my gratitude to my sisters, Ms Prerna and Mridula for their praiseworthy support during my writing.

Of course, it would be in the fitness of things to place on record the endless cooperation, patience and valuable contribution of my husband, Mr Rajendra Sharma who has been my pillar of strength throughout my writing. Sincere indebtedness is extended to him.

Finally, an expression of most special thanks to my lovely kids, Baby Gauri Sharma and Master Aaditya Sharma for their rocking forbearance during the preparation of this book.

Above all, I express my deep sense of gratitude to God Almighty for His abiding grace and blessing, which gave me strength for the successful completion of this book.

Manuscript is seldom the result of solitary effort and this one is no exception. For all those who have contributed in this task, I will always fall short in my effort to thank them. However, I will continue trying.

God Bless

Himalayani Sharma

Contents

Clinical Record Book of Medical-Surgical Nursing

Name of the Student (in Block Letters) : ....

Register No. : ....

Age and Date of Birth : ....

Year : ....

Date of Joining the Course : ....

Passport size photograph

Name and Address of the Institution : ....

....

....

....

....

Name of the Hospital/Nursing Home (where the Medical-Surgical Nursing Clinical Practice Attended) : ....

....

....

....

....

....

Signature of Student	Signature of Class Coordinator	Signature of HOD	Signature of Principal
Date:	Date:	Date:	Date:

Index

Sl. No.	Assignment	Patient name and IPD no./ward	Diagnosis/topic	Signature of faculty

Signature of HOD
Department of Medical-Surgical Nursing

Signature of Subject Coordinator

Signature of Principal

Fundamentals of Medical-Surgical Nursing

1

OBJECTIVES

After completion of this chapter, students will be able to:

- Define health, disease, illness and wellness.
- Describe the role of a medical-surgical nurse.
- Discuss the homeostatic disturbances during diseased state.
- Explain the different types of pathophysiological reactions in the human body.

INTRODUCTION

Medical-Surgical Nursing is the health promotion, health maintenance, health care, and illness care of adult patients with suspected or confirmed diagnosis of pathophysiological function. The care in this specialty is based on the knowledge derived from the amalgamation of arts and sciences, and shaped by the knowledge of nursing.

Today medical-surgical nursing is recognized as a specialty in a full-fledged manner and the focused practice areas are seen as sub-specialties like cardiovascular nursing, oncology nursing, orthopedic nursing and so on.

Irrespective of the type of health care service or setting medical-surgical nurse should be able to use the knowledge and skills with full competence and safety when providing the client care. Rapid development in technology, increase in knowledge, and transition in health care system demands medical-surgical nurse to practice the critical thinking skills to provide holistic and comprehensive patient care. To provide quality care, the nurse uses cognitive, technical, interpersonal, and ethical competencies essential to nursing profession.

Nature of Nursing

1. Nursing is caring.
2. Nursing is an art and a science.
3. Nursing is holistic.
4. Nursing is adaptive.
5. Nursing is patient centered.

Aims of Nursing

Four aims of nursing practice are:

1. To promote health
2. To prevent illness
3. To restore health
4. To facilitate coping with death and/or disability.

Who are the Recipients of Nursing

Patient: Any sick person waiting or undergoing treatment and care at a health care agency.

Society: A group of people forming a community, and receiving a health care service.

CONCEPTS IN MEDICAL-SURGICAL NURSING

Health

Health is a state of being that people define in relation to their own value, personality and lifestyle. It is also the ability to maintain roles and responsibilities.

World Health Organization (1948) defines health as 'a state of complete physical, mental, social and spiritual well-being and not merely an absence of disease or infirmity.' This is an all encompassing definition and perfectly places health on a higher pedestal in comparison to disease. This is also the most widely accepted definition among students.

Florence Nightingale states health as 'being well and using to the fullest extent every power we have.'

Illness

An illness is the response of the person to a disease. It is an abnormal process in which individual's functioning capacity is generally lowered as compared to the previous level. Illness and illness behaviour are described according to individual perception.

Disease

Disease is a medical term, meaning that there is a pathologic change in the structure or function of the body or mind. It process comprises of specific symptoms.

Always remember that an individual may have a disease but still achieve maximum functioning and quality of life.

Acute Illness

An acute illness has a rapid onset of symptoms and last for a shorter period and is self limiting in nature. Acute illness may prove fatal, some like common cold may not require any medical aid. It responds to self treatment or to medical-surgical intervention. A client with an acute illness has a full or rapid recovery. The patterns of acute illness behavior are: (i) temporary, (ii) reversible, (iii) pathology in one restricted body system, (iv) immediate short treatment plan, (v) achieving full recovery.

Chronic Illness

Chronic illness is a term that encompasses myriad lifelong pathologic or psychologic alteration in health. It includes: (i) Permanent, (ii) Nonreversible, (iii) Pathologic impairment in more than one body system, (iv) It requires long treatment plans, (v) Special rehabilitation training as well.

Disease Classification

Acute	A disease that has a rapid onset, lasts for a short time and is self-limiting, e.g. common cold
Chronic	A disease that has one or more of these characteristics (i) permanent (ii) nonreversible damage (iii) nonreversible pathophysiology (iv) require long treatment (v) special rehabilitation training, e.g. MI, CRF
Communicable	A disease that spreads from one person to another, e.g. tuberculosis, scabies
Degenerative	A disease that occurs due to deteriorating organs or tissues, e.g. osteoarthritis
Functional	A disease that affects function or performance but does not manifests any organic alteration, e.g. irritable bowel syndrome
Malignant	A disease that worsens or may cause death, e.g. cancer cervix, leukemia
Psychosomatic	A disease has a psychologic origin but has physiologic symptoms
Idiopathic	A disease whose cause is not known. A disease occurring as a result of medical therapy/ negligence, e.g. Iatrogenic pneumothorax may result from puncture of visceral pleura during central-line placement or thoracentesis, e.g. idiopathic hypertrophic subaortic stenosis, thrombocytopenia

Wellness

Wellness is a state of well being. Wellness includes self-responsibility; a dynamics and growing process Well-being is a subjected perceptionof vitality and feeling well.

Wellness is defined as being equivalent to health. It is a dynamic state of optimal health in which an individual maximizes human potential, achieving an optimal balance between internal and external environment.

It integrates physical, intellectual, sociocultural, psychological and spiritual wellness.

During the entire tenure of service nurses work to promote wellness, and prevent illness. The top level of wellness should be the goal of every nurse and client.

Prevention

Primary Prevention: Primary prevention is a true form of prevention; as it precedes disease or illness behavior. It is focused on health promotion activities such as exercise, dietary modification, immunization, health education programs as these are aimed at improving the general health of individuals, families and society at large.

Secondary Prevention: Secondary prevention focuses on individuals who have developed the disease and are at risk of developing complications or worsening conditions. It is directed at precise diagnosis and treatment and assisting the individual to resume normal level of health as early as possible.

Tertiary Prevention: Tertiary prevention is followed as a result of a disability or an irreversible damage to health. Activities at this level helps patients to achieve a higher level of functioning irrespective of the degree of disability or impairment.

Rehabilitation

Rehabilitation helps restore a person to the fullest physical, mental, social, vocational, and economic potential possible. Patients need rehabilitation after any kind of physical or mental illness or injury or substance abuse. Initial rehabilitation focuses on prevention of complications related to illness. As the patient condition improves rehabilitation helps to maximize the patient's functioning and level of independence.

GENERAL PATHOPHYSIOLOGICAL REACTIONS

Infection

Infection is the multiplication and invasion of a disease causing microorganism (pathogen) in the body tissue.

Inflammation

Inflammation is the basic pathophysiological reaction of the vascular and supporting elements of the cells or tissues which result in the formation of a protein rich exudates, and is caused by injury, provided the injury has not been so severe as to destroy the area.

Cardinal signs of inflammation are – Redness, heat, pain, swelling and exudate formation.

Atrophy

Atrophy is the reduction in size of an organ or part of it or tissues or of a single cell. Atrophy of an organ may be due to decrease in number of its structural units or in size of the individual units or both.

It may occur due to many reasons but few of them are: starvation, prolonged chronic infections, or senile changes, organ disuse.

Not always atrophy is pathologic in nature. In normal event organ atrophy takes place. Common examples are ovaries and breast atrophy after menopause.

Necrosis

Necrosis is the local death of cells without showing any signs of degeneration, still it is a part of living tissue. There is a loss of enzymatic and metabolic function. It may occur due to loss of blood supply, bacterial toxins or other factors like physical, chemical, radiation exposure.

Disturbance in Fluid, Electrolyte and Acid-Base Balance

Any kind of imbalance occurs when homeostasis mechanism is no more effective. Almost every organ and body system helps to maintain a homeostasis.

1. Acid-Base Imbalance

A respiratory disturbance alters the carbonic acid portion in the body.

Respiratory acidosis *is the excess of carbonic acid in extracellular component. Respiratory acidosis* is caused due to alveolar hypoventilation. The $PaCO_2$ increases causing an excess of carbonic acid in the blood which decreases pH. The kidneys compensate by increasing metabolic acids secretion in the urine, causing increased blood bicarbonate levels.

Respiratory alkalosis *is* the deficit of carbonic acid in the extracellular fluid. *Respiratory alkalosis* arises from alveolar hyperventilation .The lungs start excreting excess of carbonic acid (CO_2 and H_2O).The $PaCO_2$ decreases, which results in carbonic acid deficit in blood, which increases pH. Since respiratory alkalosis is mostly short lived; kidneys do not have time to compensate. If pH rises high enough CNS depression can set in. An increase in respiratory rate and depth causes CO_2 loss at a faster rate than normal.

Metabolic acidosis occurs when there is an increase in metabolic acid or a decrease of base (bicarbonate). The kidneys do not excrete enough metabolic acid which accumulates in the blood or bicarbonate is removed from the body directly as in diarrheal conditions and the HCO_3 decreases. Fall in pH stimulates the chemoreceptors so the respiratory system compensates for acidosis by hyperventilation. *Metabolic acidosis* is a proportionate deficit of bicarbonate in ECF (or acid excess) due to a gain of fixed acid or a loss of bicarbonate.

Metabolic alkalosis occurs when there is an increase in base (HCO_3). The respiratory compensation for metabolic alkalosis is hypoventilation. The decreased rate and depth of respiration causes carbonic acid levels to increase in blood and increased $PaCO_2$. *Metabolic alkalosis* is a primary excess of bicarbonate in ECF due to excessive acid losses or internal base retention.

2. Electrolyte Imbalances

Electrolyte imbalance refers to a deficit or excess of an electrolyte such as sodium, potassium, calcium, magnesium or phosphate.

Hypernatremia – Hypernatremia refers to an excess of sodium (Na) in ECF due to excessive water loss or an overall sodium excess. *Hypernatremia*, also called water deficit,is a hypertonic condition that makes body fluid too concentrated: loss of more water than salt or gain of more salt than water. It may occur in combination with extracellular volume deficit resulting in clinical dehydration. Due to increasing extracellular osmotic pressure fluid moves out of the cells.

Hyponatremia - *Hyponatremia* refers to a sodium deficit in ECF due to excessive water gain or an overall sodium loss. *Hyponatremia is*, also called water excess or water intoxication, is a hypotonic condition that makes body fluid too diluted: loss of more salt than water or gain of more water than salt. Due to increasing extracellular osmotic pressure, fluid moves out of the cells. Hyponatremia refers to a sodium deficit in ECF due to excessive water gain or an overall sodium loss. Due to increase in osmotic pressure, fluid moves in the cellular wall making it turgid.

Hyperkalemia – Hyperkalemia refers to excess potassium in ECF. *Hyperkalemia* is high potassium ion concentration in the blood. It is caused by shift of potassium from cells into the ECF, and increased potassium intake and absorption.

Hypokalemia - *Hypokalemia* is abnormally low potassium concentration in blood. This results from decreased potassium intake and absorption, and a shift of potassium from ECF into the cells. Hypokalemia can result in life- threatening weakened respiratory muscles and cardiac dysrythmias.

Skeletal muscles are the first to get affected by potassium deficit in the form of muscular weakness.

Hypercalcemia and hypocalcemia: Hypercalcemia refers to an excess of calcium in ECF. It quite often results in cardiac arrest, therefore it should be treated as an emergency. Hypocalcemia refers to a calcium deficit in ECF.

Prolonged hypocalcemia results in Ca absorption from bones resulting in osteomalacia.

Hypermagnesemia and hypomagnesemia: Hypermagnesemia refers to excess of magnesium. It is specially seen in end stage renal disease when kidneys fail to excrete magnesium. Hypomagnesemia is the deficit in magnesium levels.

Hyperphosphatemia and hypophosphatemia: Hyperphosphatemia refers to an above normal serum concentration levels of inorganic phosphorus, it causes numbness, muscle spasm, tingling. Hypophosphatemia refers to a below normal serum concentration levels of inorganic phosphorus, it can result in seizure, acute respiratory failure.

3. Fluid Imbalances

Fluid volume deficit: Fluid volume deficit can be caused due to deficiency in the amount of both water and electrolytes in the ECF. This state is called as hypovolemia or dehydration. Due to changes in osmotic and hydrostatic pressure interstitial fluid is forced into the intravascular space causing the depletion of interstitial space. The fluid now becomes hypertonic and cellular fluid is now drawn into the interstitial space leaving the cells without adequate fluid to function effectively.

Fluid volume excess: Retention of water and sodium in ECF results in fluid volume excess. This state is called as hypervolemia. Retention of sodium increases extracellular osmotic pressure.

Shock

Shock is defined as a condition of acute peripheral circulatory failure due to derangement of circulatory function. It is evidenced in the form of hypotension, cold and clammy skin, tachycardia, anxiety, and disturbed mental equilibrium.

1. **Hypovolemic shock** - Hypovolemia is encountered in sudden fluid loss through hemorrhage or the shift of fluid from vessels to the interstitial or intracellular spaces. There is reduction of effective circulatory blood volume, diminished venous return, low central venous pressure, tachycardia, reduced stroke volume, low cardiac output, drop in peripheral blood pressure and reduced oxygen delivery. If not managed it results in irreversible shock.
2. **Cardiogenic or central shock** - Any disease producing acute cardiac failure is related to this kind of situation. The basic hemodynamic defect is great loss of myocardial strength, reduction in stroke volume, cardiac output, fall in blood pressure. Compensatory mechanism is activated resulting in sympathetic vasoconstriction, increased peripheral resistance, tissue underperfusion, low urine output, elevated lactate levels, fall in blood pH. Unless this crisis is controlled, the patient goes in ever deepening shock and dies.
3. **Irreversible shock** - Whatever the type and cause of shock, unless the hemodyanamics and metabolic deterioration is controlled, there comes a stage when the patient condition is worst and is known as irreversible shock. It is evidenced by drastically reduced circulatory blood volume, resulting in tissue ischemia, acidosis, hypoxia, bacterial toxins (normally GIT contains bacterial flora) contribute to fall of arterial pressure. Damage to cellular membrane leads to leakage of lysosomal enzyme and intracellular ions and to cellular destruction.
4. **Toxic Shock Syndrome** - Toxic Shock Syndrome (TSS) is an acute condition caused by exotoxins secreted by strains of Staphylococcus aureus. TSS is characterized by fever above 102° F (38.90), hypotension, erythematous rashes, multiple organ system injury. Prompt diagnosis and treatment and antibiotic therapy is crucial.
5. **Septic Shock** - Septic shock is a state of widely disseminated infection in the bloodstream (i.e. septicemia). Initial septic shock begins with fever hypoxia, cloudy sensorium, hypotension, tachycardia, tachypnea. Treatment is with antibiotics, fluid volume replacement oxygen, diuretics, inotropic agents and heparin.
6. **Neurogenic Shock** - Loss of vasomotor tone in peripheral blood vessels leads to sudden vasodilation and pooling of blood. Vasodilation causes hypotension. Causes may be brain hemorrhage, congestive heart failure, pulmonary edema, deep anesthesia, vagal reflex and emotional trauma.

Pain

Pain is a complex, multidimensional, elusive, subjective and personal experience. 'Pain is whatever the experiencing person says it is existing whenever the person says he does'. Margo Mc Caffery, 1979).

Two basic categories of pain are generally noticed: acute pain and chronic pain.

1. **Acute pain** - Acute pain lasts from few seconds to 6 months and has an immediate onset. It is described as 'sharp' 'shooting' and 'stabbing' kind. It is controllable with adequate treatment. It is accompanied by sympathetic over activity - (i) increased or decreased blood pressure, (ii) tachycardia (iii) diaphoresis (iv) tachypnea (v) focusing on the pain and (vi) glairing the painful part. Unrelieved acute pain leads to chronic state.
2. **Chronic pain** - Chronic pain may be divided into three types:
   Chronic nonmalignant pain, e.g. rheumatoid arthritis
   Chronic intermittent pain, e.g. migraine headache
   Chronic malignant pain, e.g. cancer pain

Chronic nonmalignant pain - Chronic nonmalignant pain lasts for more than 6 months. It is continuous and recurrent in nature. It is generally associated with concomitant

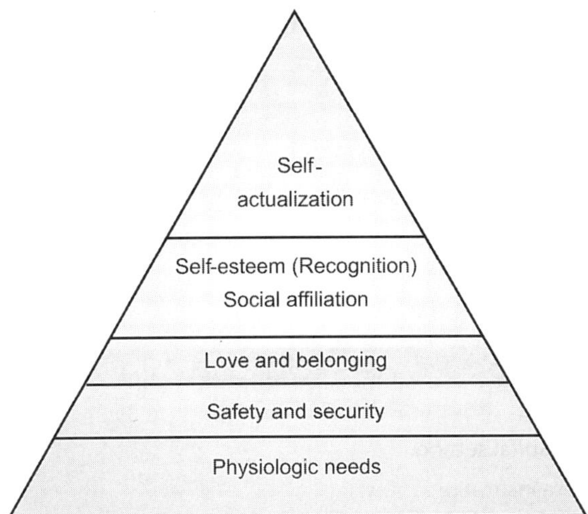

Fig. 1.1: Maslow's hierarchy of basis human needs

disability like rheumatoid arthritis in which severe pain results in restricted mobility.

Chronic intermittent pain – Chronic intermittent pain refers to exacerbation or remission of the chronic illness. This pain occurs at particular periods and at other times the client is free from pain. For example, a variation in weather conditions may aggravate a particular kind of pain.

Chronic malignant pain – Malignant pain is also called cancer-related pain. It has the quality of both the acute and chronic pain. The diagnosis of cancer adds to an increased anxiety and the potential for impending death preceded by agonizing illness.

Basic Human Needs

Human being has both the physical and psychosocial needs. Abraham Maslow (1868-1954) developed a hierarchy of basic human needs. The basic human needs in the level of priority are (Fig. 1.1):

Level 1	Physiologic needs	Breathing, temperature, food and fluid intake, circulations, sexuality, elimination, rest and mobility
Level 2	Safety and security needs	Environment, shelter, physical safety
Level 3	Love and belonging needs	Interpersonal relationship, support system, community acceptance
Level 4	Self-esteem needs	Self-acceptance, Recognition, success
Level 5	Self-actualization needs	Values, beliefs, decision making

Role of Medical-Surgical Nurse

Caregiver: As a caregiver nurse combines the art and science of nursing in providing the comprehensive care to her patients.

Communicator: Effective use of communication skills helps maintaining relationship with different kinds of patients.

Teacher: Nurse uses teaching skills to meet the learning needs of patients and their families.

Counselor: Communication skills help share information about need based referrals and develop patient's problem-solving and decision making skills.

Leader: Nurse acts as a leader by being assertive and self confident when providing care and function in/with the group.

Researcher: Being a part of any research, project broadens its knowledge base and quality nursing care.

Advocate: The nurse protects human rights of all her patients based on the fact that patients have all the rights to make informed decisions about their own health and lives.

Hospital Admission, Transfer and Discharge

2

OBJECTIVES

After completion of this chapter, students will be able to:

- Compare the client admission to an ambulatory care center and a hospital setting.
- Discuss the transfer of patients within and among various health care institutions.
- Describe the components of discharge planning that are used to provide continuity of care.
- Explain how patients are free to leave the hospital against any medical advice.

INTRODUCTION

Hospital is an integral part of social and medical organization, the function of which is to provide for the population a complete health care, both curative and preventive and whose out-patient services reach out to the family and its home environment, hospital is also a center for the training of health worker and for biosocial research (World Health Organization).

ADMISSION TO HEALTH CARE INSTITUTION

Admission to Ambulatory Care Center

Ambulatory care centers are those where the patient receives health care services from morning to evening but does not stay overnight. Admission in this kind of center is quite different. Diagnostic tests and admission procedure are completed before coming to the center. They arrive at the center, get the procedure performed and are sent home after a satisfactory recovery.

Admission to Hospital

Hospitalized patient includes those who are actually ill, victims of traumatic injuries, critically ill or those who have an acute exacerbation of a chronic disorder. Patients are admitted to a hospital in several ways.

Direct Admission

Patient is seen and examined by the physician and it is recommended that he needs special observation, monitoring and nursing care.

Emergency Admission

Emergency is a situation where the client requires immediate intervention. Here the patient is seen in an emergency department and it is determined that he needs surgery, special monitoring and nursing care.

Scheduled Admission

These are prefixed admissions where the patient opts to undergo surgery or a special diagnostic procedure that requires specialized monitoring and nursing care.

Admission to a hospital starts in the admission office, baseline information is printed on the admission sheet which is a part of patient's permanent record.

Baseline Information Collected during Hospital Admission

Full Name	Date of Admission
Address	Time of admission
Father's Name	Hospital registration No.
Age	Admission Diagnosis
Sex	
Attending physician	
Religion	

After the necessary forms have been completed, patient is shifted to the unit on wheelchair/stretcher/or walking depending on his condition.

Preparing the Room for Admission

It is the duty of an admission office to inform the unit where the patient is to be admitted so that the room can be prepared well in advance. Patient's bed, linen equipment, supplies and environment are adjusted according to his needs.

Reception and Welcome to the Unit

Patient should be welcomed and received with warmth, courtesy, and empathy. Introduction with the attending nurse and other staff members helps the client to orient them to the surroundings, ward routines, facilities available, hospital polices.

TRANSFERRING A PATIENT

Transferring refers to shifting a client from one level of care to another according to his condition. Patients are transferred within and between different levels of care to meet the varying needs and deliver the best possible care.

- Patient transfer is a common movement made within health care organization.
- Patients are transferred within the hospital, like from operation theater to recovery room, labor room to hospital room.
- Patients are transferred from acute or long-term care setting to rehabilitation centers.
- Patients are transferred from long-term settings to their homes.

In any type of transferring movement, nurse in the original area gives a detailed verbal report of her patient to the nurse in the new area. Patient's belongings are packed and shifted along with the patient.

Types of Transfer

Internal Transfer: Transferring the patient within a hospital to an advanced and specialized unit to provide care suited to his needs, e.g. ICU, recovery room.

External Transfer: Transferring the patient from one hospital to another for special care. This includes shifting the patient from general hospital to super speciality hospital.

DISCHARGE FROM A HEALTH CARE SETTING

Discharge refers to release of a patient from any health care setting to home health care facility. Discharge planning begins right at the time of admission when the data is collected and documented.

HOSPITAL ADMISSION, TRANSFER AND DISCHARGE

The purpose of discharge planning is to ensure that patient needs thoroughly met during this movement towards home health care. During the hospital stay patient should be educated about his diet medication, follow-up care, lifestyle modification. Any procedures should be demonstrated and practiced till the patient and caregivers are confident to perform them at home.

LEAVING AGAINST MEDICAL ADVICE (LAMA)

A situation in which the patient leaves the health care facility against the physician's order or his wish is known as leaving against medical advice. Although the patient has legal choice to discontinue the care, but this choice carries a risk for increasing illness or complications. Patient is required to sign the LAMA form that safeguards the physician and the health care organization from any legal responsibility for his health status. Inform the patient about any risks involved in the action being taken.

Nursing Process

3

OBJECTIVES

After completion of this chapter, students will be able to:
- Describe the nursing process and its components.
- Comprehend the significance of nursing process.
- Draw a comparison between objectives and objective database.
- Build up the skill in writing nursing care plan for their patients.
- Construct a plan of care essential to deliver a quality patient care.

NURSING PROCESS OVERVIEW

The profession of nursing has developed a pool of knowledge that leads to growth and well-being of individual and community, prevention of illness, promotion of health. The nursing process helps you to organize and deliver a pertinent nursing to a client. It is a dynamic, systematic, scientific and intellectual activity that enables you to execute care according to changing client needs.

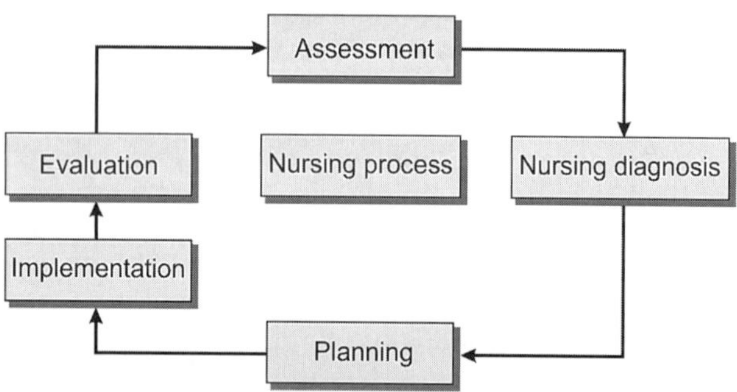

Fig. 3.1: The nursing process

The nursing process is defined as the application of critical thinking to client care activities. Traditionally, nursing process is defined as a systematic method of **assessing** health, **diagnosing** health care needs, drawing a **plan** of care, **implementing** this plan and finally **evaluating** the effectiveness of plan of care (Fig. 3.1). The use of nursing process helps the student nurses to behave as professional trained nurses. Nursing process also provides a means for evaluating the quality nursing care delivered by nurses and assures their accountability to the consumers. It provides a framework that helps nurse and patient to accomplish the following:

- Systematic data collection (assess)
- Identify patient strengths and actual or potential problem (diagnose)
- Develop an individual need based plan of care, clearly specifying the desired goals and outcomes and nursing interventions helping the client to achieve these expected outcomes (plan)
- Execute the plan of care (intervening)
- Evaluate the effectiveness of administered care in term of goal achievement (evaluating).

I THE ASSESSMENT STEP: DEVELOPING THE PATIENT DATABASE

Assessment is the first step of Nursing process. This must be pertinent to the client's particular health problem. Assessment aims at organizing the database related to the patient's physical, psychosocial and emotional health so as to identify health promoting behavior.

Information collected through assessment can be subjective data and objective data.

Subjective data are the client's (sometimes significant others) perceptions about their health problems. This data can only be reported by the client and is collected through an interview.

Objective data are the observations and measurements made by the nurse by performing physical examination, reports of various investigation findings.

II NURSING DIAGNOSIS: ANALYZING THE DATA

Nursing diagnosis is the second step of nursing process. This step gives meaning and direction to the data collected during the assessment phase. The terms Analysis/Problem/Need Identification or Nursing Diagnosis are used interchangeably.

According to NANDA (The North American Nursing Diagnosis Association) 'Nursing Diagnosis is a clinical judgment about individual, family or community responses to actual and potential health problems/life processes. Nursing diagnosis provides the basis for selection of nursing intervention to achieve outcomes for which the nurse is accountable'.

The Use of Nursing Diagnosis

- Gives nurses a common language.
- Promotes identification of appropriate goals.
- Can create a standard nursing practice.
- Provides a quality improvement base.

NANDA Nursing Diagnosis Taxonomy II

Activity intolerance	Coping, compromised family	Grieving, dysfunction
Activity intolerance, risk for	Coping, defensive	Growth and development, delayed
Adjustment, impaired	Coping, disabled family	Growth, risk for disproportionate
Airway clearance, ineffective	Coping, ineffective	Health maintenance, ineffective
Allergy response, latex	Coping, ineffective community	Health-seeking behaviors
Allergy response, risk for latex	Coping, readiness for enhanced community	Home maintenance, impaired
Anxiety	Coping, readiness for enhanced family	Hopelessness
Anxiety, death	Denial, ineffective	Hyperthermia
Aspiration, risk for	Dentition, impaired	Hypothermia
Attachment, risk for impaired parent/infant/child	Development, risk for delayed	Identity, disturbed personal
Autonomic dysreflexia	Diarrhea	Incontinence, functional
Autonomic dysreflexia, risk for	Disuse syndrome, risk for	Incontinence, reflex urinary
Body image, disturbed	Diversional activity, deficient	Incontinence, stress urinary
Body temperature, risk for imbalanced	Energy field, disturbed	Incontinence, total urinary
Bowel incontinence	Environmental interpretation syndrome, impaired	Incontinence, urge urinary
Breastfeeding, effective	Failure to thrive, adult	Incontinence, risk for urge urinary
Breastfeeding, ineffective	Falls, risk for	Infant behavior, disorganized
Breastfeeding, interrupted	Family processes, dysfunctional; alcoholism	Infant behavior, readiness for enhanced organized
Breathing pattern, ineffective	Family processes, interrupted	Infant feeding pattern, ineffective
Cardiac output, decreased	Fatigue	Infection, risk for
Caregiver role strain, risk for	Fear	Injury, risk for
Comfort, impaired	Fluid volume, deficient	Injury, risk for perioperative-positioning
Communication, impaired verbal	Fluid volume, excess	Intracranial adaptive capacity, decreased
Conflict, decisional	Fluid volume, risk for deficient	Knowledge, deficient
Conflict, parental role	Fluid volume, risk for imbalanced	Loneliness, risk for
Confusion, acute	Gas exchange, impaired	Memory, impaired
Confusion, chronic	Grieving	Mobility, impaired bed
Constipation	Grieving, anticipatory	Mobility, impaired physical
Constipation, perceived		Mobility, impaired wheelchair
Constipation, risk for		Nausea

Contd...

Contd...

Neglect, unilateral	Relocation stress syndrome, risk for	Suffocation, risk for
Noncompliance	Role performance, ineffective	Suicide, risk for
Nutrition, imbalanced: Less than body requirements	Self-care deficit, bathing/hygiene	Surgical recovery, delayed
	Self-care deficit, dressing/grooming	Swallowing, impaired
Nutrition, imbalanced: More than body requirements	Self-care deficit, feeding	Therapeutic regimen management, effective
	Self-care deficit, toileting	
Nutrition, risk imbalanced: More than body requirements	Self-esteem, chronic low	Therapeutic regimen management, ineffective
Oral mucous membrane, impaired	Self-esteem, situational low	Therapeutic regimen management, ineffective community
Pain, acute	Self-esteem, risk for situational low	
Pain, chronic	Self-mutilation	Therapeutic regimen ineffective family
Parenting, impaired	Self-mutilation, risk for	Thermoregulation, ineffective
Parenting, risk for impaired	Sensory perception, disturbed	Thought processes, disturbed
Peripheral neurovascular dysfunction, risk for	Sexual dysfunction	Tissue integrity, impaired
	Sexuality patterns, ineffective	Tissue perfusion, ineffective
Poisoning, risk for	Skin integrity, impaired	Transfer ability, impaired
Post-trauma syndrome	Skin integrity, risk for impaired	Trauma, risk for
Post-trauma syndrome, risk for	Sleep deprivation	Urinary elimination, impaired
Powerlessness	Sleep pattern, disturbed	Urinary retention
Powerlessness, risk for	Social interaction, impaired	Ventilation, impaired spontaneous
Protection, ineffective	Social isolation	Ventilatory weaning response, dysfunctional
Rape-trauma syndrome	Sorrow, chronic	
Rape-trauma syndrome: Compound reaction	Spiritual distress	Violence, risk for other-directed
	Spiritual distress, risk for	Violence, risk for self-directed
Rape-trauma syndrome: Silent reaction	Spiritual well-being, readiness for enhanced	Walking, impaired
Relocation stress syndrome		Wandering

From North American Nursing Diagnosis Association: NANDA nursing diagnosis: definitions, and classification, 2001-2002, Philadelphia, 2001, The Association.

III THE PLANNING STEP: CREATING THE PLAN OF CARE

Once the nursing diagnosis statements have been finalized you can proceed to the planning step of nursing process. Here, attention is focused on the actions which are most appropriate to address the patient problems. The nurse begins to set priority, establish goals, identify desired outcomes and determine specific nursing interventions.

Once the patient problems have been prioritized establish the goals of treatment. Goals may be long-term or short term. Long-term goals indicate the end result of care and may not be achieved before discharge. Short-term goals are more specific guidelines for care and must usually be met before discharge or transfer to a less acute level of care.

Identifying Desired Outcomes

Specific outcomes are defined as patient responses that are realistic, specific, measurable and achievable within a definite time frame. Measurable action verbs are used to describe outcomes. Properly written outcomes provide direction for planning and validating the choice of nursing intervention.

Selecting appropriate Nursing Interventions

Nursing interventions are prescriptions for behavior, treatment activities or actions that assist the patient in achieving the expected outcomes. To be accurate nursing interventions, need to be developed in the correct format and be specifically and clearly stated. Follow the criteria while documenting the intervention in the patient's plan of care.

- The date when the intervention is written
- The action verb describing the activity
- Time, frequency, where and amount
- Signature of the attending nurse.

IV THE IMPLEMENTATION STEP: ACTING UPON THE PLAN OF CARE

Implementation refers to the 'hands-on' phase of nursing process. It is the actual initiation of plan and recording of nursing actions. It aims at providing technical and therapeutic nursing care required to help the client achieve set goals.

Before implementing the interventions listed in the plan of care, you need to be sure that you:

- Understand the rationale for carrying out the intervention, its expected effect and any potential hazards that can occur.
- Provide an environment conducive to carrying out the planned intervention.
- Consider which interventions can be combined so you can accomplish the activities within your time constraints.

V THE EVALUATION STEP: DETERMINING IF DESIRED OUTCOMES HAVE BEEN MET

Evaluation, the final step of nursing process is defined as the judgment of the effectiveness of nursing care to meet client goals based on his behavioral response. Evaluation is an ongoing process which is necessary for determining how well the plan of care is working. Evaluation step has three components:

- Reassessment
- Modification of the plan of care
- Termination of services.

Reassessment

Reassessment is a constant 'measuring and monitoring' of the patient's status that looks at the patient's response to nursing interventions and progress toward attaining the desired outcome. Evaluating the data determines:

- The appropriateness of nursing actions
- The need to revise the interventions
- The development of new patient needs.

Modification of the Plan of Care

Upon evaluating the outcomes and the plan of care, nurse may find that the patient's condition has changed in a direction which was not anticipated regardless of her nursing intervention, at this point a change in treatment approach/plan of care is indicated.

As the plan of care is modified, remember to address the changing needs of patient, environment, and therapeutic regimen. At this stage, a patient care conference may be scheduled with other members of health team to provide problem-solving solutions.

Termination of Care

When the desired outcomes have been achieved and the broader goals met, termination of care is planned. Even though the patient has been discharged it is important for the patient and family to know what has been achieved and how they can continue to enhance patient further health status. Discharge summary must be discussed to promote continuity of care.

Criteria for Writing the Nursing Care Plan

There are various methods of writing a nursing care plan and it may vary from institution to institution. In this record book, we are using a format that has all the basic components of nursing process:

- Assessment
- Nursing diagnosis
- Goals—Short-term and long-term
- Nursing interventions
- Outcomes
- Status of objectives.

4

Health Assessment

OBJECTIVES

After completion of this chapter, students will be able to:

- Develop a broad knowledge based on physical health assessment.
- Explain the concept of patient and environmental preparation for health assessment.
- Identify and utilize the techniques involved in physical assessment.
- Conduct a physical examination in proper systematic manner.
- Develop a skill to collect a detailed health history of a patient.

INTRODUCTION

Health assessment is a vital component of nursing process. It is the health assessment around which entire nursing care is directed. Nurses are employed in different health settings, seeking baseline information about client's health status. A thorough health assessment involves a detailed health history and physical examination. A physical examination is a head-to-toe review of all body system that provides objective data. The health history is a detailed and patient interview to obtain subjective data.

PHYSICAL EXAMINATION

Physical examination is the systematic, organized, superficial check of body systems to detect any abnormality or problems. It is performed following a detailed health history interview. Collect objective data to supplement and validate subjective data so that both can be evaluated to assess holistic perception of the client.

Techniques of Physical Examination

There are four sequential techniques of physical examinations.

a. Inspection (1st technique)
   Inspection is the systematic, visual examination of body surface area. It provides information about size, shape, color, texture, symmetry, position and deformity.
b. Palpation (2nd technique)
   Palpation is the use of touch by exerting variable degree of pressure to gather information about any masses, pulsation, tenderness, swelling and temperature. The degree of pressure applied during palpation varies. This is done slowly and gently.
c. Percussion (3rd technique)
   Percussion is used to assess tissue density by generation of sound by striking over the body surface. It is done by placing a finger of the left hand firmly against the part to be examined and tapping with right hand fingers. The sounds heard upon percussion could be following:
   Resonance: A low pitch and loud sound heard over the normal lung tissues.
   Hyperresonance: Very loud, very low pitch sound longer than resonance and is of booming nature is a sign of COPD.
   Tympany: A drum like sound heard over the air filled tissues like gastric air bubble.
   Dull: A medium pitched sound of a medium duration without resonance heard over solid organs like liver.
   Flat: A high pitched sound with a short duration without resonance heard over complete solid organs like hand, thighs.
d. Auscultation (4th technique)
   Auscultation is the final step of physical examination. It is the technique of listening to normal body sounds and differentiating them from abnormal sounds. It is done by using a stethoscope.
e. Manipulation
   Manipulation is the moving of a part of the body to note its flexibility. Restricted movements are noted by this method.

Recording and Reporting

Record the findings of physical examination in the patient file. Use accurate, appropriate and descriptive glossary as it forms a foundation for future physical findings.

GUIDELINES FOR HEALTH HISTORY INTERVIEW

Assessment of the client provides basic data for the nursing process. Assessment provides verification and identification of physical and psychosocial needs. Health assessment focuses on the client and has several parts. Health history provides subjective and objective information.

1. **Patient preparation**
   - Introduce yourself, and explain the purpose of interview.
   - Talk softly, calmly, and patiently.
   - Begin with nonprobing, client-centered question and proceed towards focused questions to identify, problem areas.
   - Observe for any discomfort in facial expressions and/or body language.
2. **Environmental preparation**
   - Select a room with comfortable setting (providing privacy)
   - Eliminate any distractions (TV, radio)
   - Maintain moderate room temperature (degree of seasonal cooling/heating)
   - Adjust indirect lighting to prevent dazzling that may affect communication.
3. **Preparation of interviewer**
   - Avoid repetitive questioning. Follow a structured but flexible format.
   - Inform your patient about noting down the information gathered.
   - Follow termination of interview by summarizing and permitting the client for clarification of any doubts.

Components of Health History

Health history assessment can be organized and made more informative by putting into a structured format that provides a tool for collecting a comprehensive data.

HEALTH ASSESSMENT FORMAT
Nursing History and Physical Examination

Date:

Place:

History:

i. Biographic and/or demographic details

Name: Age: Sex: M/F

Address:

Permanent:

____

____

Present:

____

____

Hospital registration no: ________________

Date of admission: ________________

Ward and unit: ________________

Bed no: ________________

Marital status: ________________

Religion: ________________

Language: ________________

Educational qualifications: ________________

Occupation: ________________

*Name of the attendant/family members ________________

Age: ________________

* The information is collected from a close reliable family member

Relationship with the client: ____________________

Address: ____________________

Diagnosis:

ii. Patient's reason for hospitalization

____

iii. History of present illness

(Provide the details in chronological order specifying the symptoms, onset, duration, precipitating factors, relief measures adopted).

____

iv. Past health history

____

- Past illness history

____

- Treatment – surgical/medical/any other

____

- Details of previous hospitalization

____

- Allergies

____

- Menstruation

  Age at menarchy ____________________

  Regular/irregular ____________________

  LMP ____________________

  Menopause ____________________

- Details of immunization

____

- Personal habits

____

- Current medication being taken

____

- Sleeping pattern (regular/irregular/any sleep disorder)

____

- Any fitness/exercise pattern

____

- Dietary details : Vegetarian/Non-vegetarian/egg-vegetarian/Special diet ______
- Job/Work details : Any shifts/Sitting or standing

______

______

v. Family history (make a family tree in the space provided and write the details)

- History of any chronic illness: (DM, HTN, CAD, any other) ______
- History of any communicable disease in the family ______
- Birth/death in family

______

vi. Environmental history

- Drinking water supply ______
- Environmental sanitation ______
- Waste/excreta disposal ______
- Presence of flies/mosquitoes/rodents ______

vii. Psychosocial history

- Language ______
- Details of milestones development ______
- Social support available or not ______

SYSTEMIC PHYSICAL EXAMINATION

i. Head

Headache ______ Convulsions/seizures ______

Injury ______

ii. Eyes

Glasses/contact lens ______ Blurred vission ______

Pain ______ Inflammation ______

Watering/Discharge ______

iii. Ears

Hearing impairment ______ Hearing aid ______

Pain ______ Discharge ______

Tinnitus ______ Vertigo ______

Surgery ______

iv. Nose

Discharge ______ URI ______

Polyp ______ Epistaxis ______

Allergies ______ Sinusitis ______

Surgery ______

v. Throat and mouth

Dysphagia ______ Bleeding ______

Dental caries ______ Lesions ______

Halitosis ______ Speech disorder ______

Pain ______ Flourosis ______

Oral hygiene ______

vi. Respiratory

Cough ____________________ Sputum ____________________

Dyspnea ____________________ Dyspnea on exertion ____________________

Activity intolerance ____________________ Hemoptysis ____________________

Surgery ____________________

vii. Circulation

Pain ____________________ Palpitation ____________________

Edema ____________________ Numbness ____________________

Change in color ____________________ Syncope ____________________

Dizziness ____________________ Paroxysmal nocturnal dyspnea ____________________

Dyspnea ____________________ Postural hypotension ____________________

viii. Nutritional

Appetite ____________________ Nausea ____________________

Vomiting ____________________ Dysphagia ____________________

Indigestion ____________________ Weight change: Loss/gain ____________________

Regurgitation ____________________

ix. Elimination: Normal bowel/bladder pattern ____________________

Constipation ____________________ Diarrhea ____________________

Incontinence ____________________ Infection ____________________

Melena ____________________ Hematuria ____________________

Any surgery ____________________ Presence of catheter ____________________

x. Reproductive

No. of pregnancy ____________________ No. of live issues ____________________

Bleeding ____________________ Vaginal discharge ____________________

Infection ____________________ Pain ____________________

Nocturnal emission ____________________ Abortion ____________________

Any surgery ____________________

xi. Neurological

Confusion ____________________ Convulsions ____________________

Weakness ____________________ Loss of strength ____________________

Paralysis ____________________ Change in sensation ____________________

Incoordination ____________________ Headache ____________________

Tingling/Pricking ____________________ Pain ____________________

Memory ____________________ Numbness ____________________

Consciousness ____________________ Reflexes (specify weak reflexes) ____________________

xii. Musculoskeletal system

Pain ____________________ Joint stiffness/swelling ____________________

Joint movement ____________________ Muscle strength ____________________

Posture ____________________ Gait ____________________

Weakness ____________________ Changes in ADL ____________________

Immobility ____________________

xiii. Skin

Rashes ________________ Lesions ________________

Pallor ________________ Texture ________________

Temperature ________________ Color ________________

Nevi pigmentation ________________ Dryness ________________

xiv. Endocrinal

Any hormonal problem (Please specify)

____

____

____

xv. Hepatic system

Scleral yellowing ________________ Urinary yellowing ________________

Skin color ________________ Substance abuse ________________

Diagnostic Test

5

OBJECTIVES

After completion of this chapter, students will be able to:

- Identify the basic and advanced diagnostic tests.
- Explain the concept of patient preparation related to the test.
- Explain nursing responsibilities before, during and after the diagnostic tests.

A precise diagnosis is the corner-stone of treatment. It is the physician who formulates the diagnosis after elucidating all the facts. The nurse's observation is of great importance, over a period of time when the patient shows some improvement in his condition.

DIAGNOSTIC EVALUATION

Diagnostic evaluation refers to a variety of tests that are conducted to detect and evaluate the nature and extent of disease. These tests can vary from simple to advanced type. These tests have been classified under different headings for better understanding by students.

MICROBIOLOGICAL STUDIES

Many study types are performed to identify disease causing microbes and decide the treatment. Different types of tests are performed to identify the microorganism:

- A *smear* is the spreading of a specimen on the surface of glass slide.
- A *stain* is the application of dyes like methylene blue or basic fuchsin to identify the microorganism.
- A *culture* is the colonization of microbes on the culture plates to facilitate their growth over a period of time.
- *Sensitivity studies* are performed to determine the type of antibiotic that would impede the growth of organism.

Wet preparation: Wet preparations are also called unstained preparations. These are examined mainly for bacterial motility (e.g. hanging drop preparation) and spirochetes (dark ground microscopy).

COLLECT ALL SPECIMEN USING ASEPTIC TECHNIQUE

Culture

Culture growth allows exact identification of microbes .This method is used to determine the sensitivity of etiological agents to chemotherapeutic drugs.

Blood culture: Bacteremia is the presence of bacteria in the blood stream. A series of three blood specimen are drawn (at 30 minutes) following a strict sterile technique.

Wound culture: Material from inside a wound is procured with a sterile swab enclosed in a culture tube.

Urine culture: A clean-catch (midstream) specimen is collected in a sterile container. Urine C+S tests are performed to confirm urinary tract infections.

Stool culture: Fecal material is obtained over a sterile rectal swab to identify the type of bacteria.

Throat (swab) culture: Use a wooden spatula to depress the tongue and swab the sterile applicator with the exudates, ulceration on the throat surface.

Sputum culture: Sputum culture are collected to diagnose most of the respiratory conditions like pneumonia, emphysema, tuberculosis. This method incubates the specimen for presence of organisms. A deeply coughed out specimen must be collected for investigation.

BLOOD STUDIES

Blood can be collected by venipuncture, arterial puncture, central lines and microcapillary collection techniques. A large number of tests are performed on a blood sample.

Type and cross match: Blood types are classified as positive or negative depending upon the presence or absence of rhesus (Rh) factor. Cross match helps to determine the compatibility between a potential donor and recipient.

URINE STUDIES

Urinalysis: Urinalysis is one of the very common laboratory tests. Normal urinalysis findings help rule out a number of alternative diagnosis. Urinalysis data include color, specific gravity, pH and presence of proteins, RBCs, WBCs, bacteria, bilirubin, urobilirubin, glucose-ketone bodies, casts and crystals.

STOOL TESTS

Stool specimen is tested for urobilinogen, occult blood, bacterial parasites, fats, ova, and fecal leucocytes.

PAPANICOLAOU TEST

A papanicolaou test (or a Pap smear) is the examination of staining exfoliative cells to evaluate the metabolic activity, cellular differentiation, maturity, and morphological variation of cervical tissue.

ELECTRODIAGNOSTIC STUDIES

Electrodiagnostic tests are performed to measure the electrical action of organs like heart, muscles, brain.

Electrodes are placed at certain body points to measure the electrical impulses which spread outward from the visceral organs to the skin.

Electrocardiography

An electrocardiogram (ECG/EKG) is a noninvasive, graphical representation of heart's electrical activity. Electrocardiography helps detect and amplify the very small electrical potential changes at different points of the body surface as the myocardial cells depolarize and repolarize, causing the heart to contract. The same electrical impulses spread outward from the heart to the skin where they get detected by the electrodes placed over the skin. The ECG displays the electrical action of the heart.

Electroencephalography

Electroencephalography (EEG) is a noninvasive, graphical recording of electrical activity of the brain. Electrodes are attached to the client's scalp, and ear lobe. The waves are amplified and recorded on a moving paper strip as for an ECG. Electroencephalography is performed to assess seizure disorder.

Electromyography

Electromyography (EMG) helps to measure and document electrical currents produced by the skeletal muscles called muscle action potential. The electrical potentials of each muscle are amplified, transmitted to an oscilloscope and visualized on a screen. The findings are documented on a paper. This test helps to identify a primary muscle disease.

Electroretinography

Electroretinography (ERG) measures the change in the electrical potential of the eye caused by a diffuse flash of light.

Electrodes incorporated into the contact lens are placed on the anesthetized eye. Retina being a neurologic tissue exhibits its electrical response when subjected to a source of light.

Electrocochleography

Electrocochleography is a test performed to measure the response of the cochlea and eighth cranial nerve to acoustic stimulation. Electrodes are placed through the tympanic membrane onto the promontory near the round window or in the ear canal and an acoustic stimulation is applied.

Stress Test/Exercise Electrocardiogram

Stress testing is defined as body's reaction to a measured increase in acute exercises. It measures and evaluates the cardiovascular conditioning and functioning by showing the myocardium's ability to respond to increased oxygen requirements by increasing the blood flow to coronary artery. The test helps to evaluate the cardiovascular parameters.

Patient is asked to walk on a treadmill which has a conveyor belt that reaches speed of 1 to 10 miles per hour, allowing the client to walk or run on varying slopes or angles. During the test continuous ECG and BP monitoring is done by a physician.

Echocardiography

Echocardiography is a noninvasive diagnostic procedure to evaluate the structural and functional changes in heart. The test is performed by placing a transducer on various areas of the chest wall. A burst of ultrasound waves are directed at particular part of heart under investigation. An echocardiogram records the structure and motion of that area in relation to its distance from the anterior chest wall, continuous ECG is recorded in a graph and images are recorded in a video tape for analysis.

Thallium Test—Thallium 201 Scintigraphy

Thallium 201 is a most widely used radioactive isotope that emits gamma rays. Thallium 201 (^{201}Tl) is an analog of potassium that is easily extracted by smooth skeletal and cardiac muscle fibers. During the test ^{201}Tl is administered intravenously. The client is asked to exercise for the last minute to ensure ^{201}Tl distribution to the heart during maximum stress (85%). The client then cools down and reclines on an examination table for perfusion scan. Continuous imaging in a 180° arc over the chest is performed. After 3 hours a repeat ^{201}Tl by IV route is injected and repeated images are taken. Two sets of images are then compared and evaluated.

DIAGNOSTIC IMAGING

Radiography

Radiography is the most noninvasive painless test for the study of bones and soft tissues. Radiography, also called an 'X-ray', is an image of a negative on photographic film obtained by exposing the film to X-rays which passes through the body.

X-ray tests are used to (a) establish the presence of mobility or anatomical problems (b) follow the progress in recovery (c) evaluate treatment interventions.

Chest X-ray Studies

Chest X-ray studies provide information about chest cavity. Chest X-ray studies are performed with the client standing or sitting facing the X-ray film and in direct contact with film cassette. This test is performed to diagnose respiratory disorders.

Chest X-rays are obtained from different views/positions to assess the entire rib cage. Remove all under clothes and metallic jewellery as it may obstruct the view of the tissue beneath. Also collect information about pregnancy status.

Skeletal X-ray

Skeletal X-rays are ordered for bones in question. Generally procedure is painless but the movement of fractured bone may cause pain to the client.

Fluoroscopy

Fluoroscopy is a radiographic procedure that allows direct visualization of the body. The body part to be examined is placed between an X-ray tube and a fluorescent screen. X-rays pass through the body and help visualize the targeted organs and/or bones on the fluoroscopic screen.

Tomography

Tomography is a radiographic technique that produces images of body tissues in a single plane or section. Serial images are clicked by moving the X-ray tube which in turn projects views at varying ends of tissue depth.

Contrast X-ray Studies

Contrast X-ray study is a radiographic technique using radiopaque media to enhance visualization of an organ system or tissue under study.

Barium Swallow: Barium swallow is a radiologic visualization of upper GIT (esophagus, stomach, duodenum, and jejunum). About 10 ounce of barium, a radiopaque contrast medium is drunk by a client who is then asked to stand before a fluoroscopy tube for visualization.

Barium Enema: Barium enema is the visualization of lower GIT. In this technique barium is instilled readily and radiographs are obtained with or without fluoroscopy.

Computed Tomography

Computed tomography (CT) is the radiological scanning of the body from radiation source. Multidimensional images of the viscera are transmitted to computer. Images are obtained by computerized synthesis of X-ray data in transverse, sagittal and coronal planes. CT scan could be plane or with contrast medium in which dye may be administered. This test generally takes 15-20 minutes to perform.

Bronchoscopy

Bronchoscopy is an X-ray test to visualize the trachea, bronchi, and entire bronchial tree after radiopaque iodine contrast is injected through a catheter into the tracheobronchial space. The bronchi gets lined with the injected dye and a series of tests are taken then. The test is done to diagnose bronchial obstruction like tumor, foreign body, cyst.

Magnetic Resonance Imaging

Magnetic resonance imaging (MRI) is a noninvasive test in which images are obtained by the use of powerful magnetic fields and radiofrequency pulses, thereby protecting the client against exposing to ionizing radiations. The magnet inside the equipment/scanner is 30,000 times stronger than the earth's magnetic field, due to which the test cannot be performed on clients with fixed devices like pacemakers, metal implants, etc.

Positron Emission Tomography

Positron emission tomography is an advance test that produces images of metabolic and physiologic functions of body. The client is given doses of radioactive tracers (radionuclide) which emit signals to show their uptake or distribution. Images are obtained by computer analysis of photons detected by annihilation of positrons emitted by radionuclides.

Angiography

Angiography is a radiographic technique that uses a contrast agent/dye to assess the anatomy of blood vessels and the flow of blood through them. This test makes use of fluoroscopy technique as well. Using fluoroscopy, the catheter is threaded through a peripheral artery into the area to be studied like coronary, pulmonary, renal, femoral, popliteal artery. Dye is injected through this vascular catheter and films are obtained in sequence. The term arteriography and angiography are used interchangeably.

Venography: Study of veins using angiography technique.

Lymphography: Study of lymphatic vessels using angiography technique.

Ultrasonography

Ultrasonography, also called an ultrasound or echogram or sonogram, is a noninvasive test that uses high frequency sound waves to study deeper body tissues. The test works on the principle of sonar or radar. The transducer directs the ultrasound waves towards the body and they spread through the tissues which are reflected back and recorded as images and photographs on the oscilloscope. No special preparation is required for this test. Inform the patient that the procedure is painless and quick to perform. A lubricating gel is placed on the body surface to increase the contact between the skin and the transducer.

Radionuclide Imaging

Radionuclide imaging or nuclear scanning uses radioisotopes or tracers to visualize body structures. Various isotopes like thallium, technetium are used because of their concentrating ability in body organs or body fluid. Radionuclide is administered orally or intravenously about 1 to 3 hours before the test to allow the time for distribution. However, blocking agent may be administered before a radionuclide to prevent uptake by certain tissues. A scintigraphic scanner, placed above the area under study, detects emitted radiations and produces a visual image.

ENDOSCOPY

Endoscopy is the direct visualization of body cavity by means of a lighted, flexible tube, called an endoscope. An endoscope is inserted directly into the body cavity to be examined. An endoscope has a well fitted light source and a camera at one end which helps the examiner to assess and visualize the lesions, any growth or anatomical defects if any.

Arthroscopy, bronchoscopy, GIT endoscopy-colonoscopy, sigmoidoscopy are a few examples of this technique.

BIOPSY/CYTOLOGIC STUDIES

Biopsy is defined as the excision of a part of a tissue.

Aspiration is the withdrawal of an abnormally collected fluid from the body cavity.

Biopsy has an important role in confirming various types of cancers. Technically biopsy is of two types—open and closed.

Open Biopsy

This technique involves giving an incision to obtain a tissue. There are two types:

1. **Excision biopsy**: The entire lesion or the border of adjacent normal tissues are removed.
2. **Incision biopsy**: A part of the lesion is removed. The procedure is done in conjunction with endoscopic examination.

Closed Biopsy

In closed biopsy, no surgical incision is given rather specially created biopsy needle with stylet is used to penetrate the skin. Once the needle is placed, stylet is withdrawn and the fluid/tissues is aspirated for examination. Different types of closed biopsy are:

- Needle aspiration biopsy—inserted into the tissue. Aspirated cells are examined.
- Core needle biopsy—a special tru-cut needle cuts the tissue from the viscera. Example is biopsy of liver and kidney.
- Punch biopsy—in this specimen is obtained by directly piercing the organ or through the skin, e.g. biopsy of skin, cervix.

Various biopsy/aspiration procedures are as follows:

- Paracentesis—is the aspiration of fluid from the peritoneal cavity. The test is performed for both the diagnostic or therapeutic purposes.
- Bone marrow aspiration—sternum and iliac crest are the bones of choice to aspirate bone marrow for diagnostic purpose.
- Thoracentesis—fluid is aspirated from pleural cavity which otherwise gets increased due to inflammation, infection, some trauma.
- Lumbar puncture/spinal tap—is the aspiration of cerebrospinal fluid from the subarachnoid space at L_3-L_4 level.
- Arthrocentesis—is the aspiration of synovial fluid from the knee joint. Biopsy needle is injected into the joint space to obtain the fluid. Anti-inflammatory drugs are also injected through this procedure for therapeutic purpose.

Lung Biopsy: Lung biopsy is an invasive procedure to obtain a specimen of pulmonary tissue for histological examination by using any of the open or closed technique. Patient is kept NPO after midnight. Open lung biopsy is performed in operation room by making an incision into the chest wall.

PULMONARY FUNCTION TEST

Pulmonary function test or PFT is done with a spirometer that measures the amount of air a patient can inhale or exhale. The test is performed in pulmonary function laboratory. It helps measure total volume, inspiratory reserve volume, expiratory reserve volume, and residual volume. Since patients get exhausted due to deep inhaling and exhaling exercise, provide rest periods in between.

ELECTROENCEPHALOGRAM

Electroencephalogram (EEG) is a noninvasive test in which electrodes are paced over the skull at various locations and electrical activity of brain segments is recorded. EEG is a painless test to rule out brain tumors, abscess seizure disorder. This test measures the electrical potential from neuron activity in the form of wave patterns. Four types of wave patterns like alpha, beta, theta and delta are studied to demonstrate wakeful, sleep, stressed and drowsy state.

ARTERIAL BLOOD GAS ANALYSIS

Arterial blood gas (ABG) analysis reveals sensitive information about acid-base balance, ventilator ability, oxygen saturation, partial pressure of oxygen and carbon dioxide. ABG is done by performing an arterial puncture.
Normal values of ABG are:

- pH:7.35 to 7.45
- pCO_2 : 35 to 45 mm Hg
- $pHCO_3$: 21 to 28mEq/L
- pO_2: 80 to 100 mm Hg
- SaO_2: 95 to 100%

THORACENTESIS

Thoracentesis is puncturing the chest wall by introducing a hollow needle into pleural cavity for removing pleural fluid and/or air. Specimen is obtained under strict aseptic technique. As the fluid or air is removed an immediate relief in respiratory stress can be witnessed. Common site for thoracentesis is just below the scapular 7th or 8th intercostals space. Maintain an upright position during the procedure as it helps to collect the fluid at the base of pleural cavity.

COMMON NURSING RESPONSIBILITIES

Before Diagnostic Test

- Monitor vital signs to establish baseline data.
- Review the client's record for any allergic reaction and signed consent form for the procedure.
- Any particular medications to be administered.
- Maintain NPO status if required for the test.
- Start IV line if required.
- Inform the client and family about the reason, duration and what to expect from the test.

During the Diagnostic Test

- Encourage deep breathing exercise to make the client comfortable while the procedure is going on.
- Check client's medical record for any specific information related to any allergy.
- Provide comfortable position.
- Follow strict aseptic technique for any invasive procedure.
- Be with the client during induction or maintenance of anesthesia.
- Keep emergency trolley ready in case of any emergency.
- Assist the physician in collection and labeling the obtained specimen.
- Monitor client's vital signs thoroughly.
- Record the procedure details in terms of performing physician, indication for procedure, anesthesia used, vital signs, any complications, specimen obtained, client's stability status.

After Diagnostic Test

- Send the specimen with complete details to the concerned lab.
- Assess vital signs and pain at the site of procedure.
- Notify the physician for any respiratory distress or untoward bleeding.
- Provide safe and comfortable position to promote patient comfort.
- Inform the physician about the results of the diagnostic findings.
- Inform the client and family for any restrictions related to diet, head elevation, activity resumption, etc.
- Record the information related to vital signs, laboratory findings, instruction given, and any drug administration.

6 Perioperative Nursing

OBJECTIVES

After completion of this chapter, students will be able to:

- Explain the concept of perioperative nursing.
- Design a preoperative teaching plan.
- Assist the patient for physical and psychological preparation for surgery.
- Utilize the nursing process to develop an individualized plan of care for surgical patient during different phases of perioperative period.

PERIOPERATIVE NURSING

Perioperative period: The entire surgical event is a perioperative period. This period includes the nursing care given before, during and after the surgery. The perioperative period consists of three phases: 1. Preoperative phase, 2. Intraoperative phase, 3. Postoperative phase.

Perioperative nursing: Perioperative nursing refers to the role of nurse during the preoperative, intraoperative and postoperative phase of patient's surgical experience. Perioperative nursing care emphasizes the importance of continuity of care.

Classification of Surgical Procedure

A broad classification of surgical procedures, depending upon the degree of seriousness, urgency and purposes is given in the Table 6.1.

Table 6.1: Classification of Surgical procedure

Type	*Description*	*Example*
Seriousness		
Major	Consists of elaborate reconstruction or alteration in body parts	Lobectomy, colostomy
Minor	Consists of minimal alteration in body parts	Tooth extraction
Urgency		
Elective	Planned procedures performed according to client's choice	Cesarean section Breast reconstruction
Urgent	Must be performed to prevent further aggravation in condition	Coronary artery bypass grafting (CABG)
Emergency	Must be performed immediately to save life or to maintain the function of body part	Appendectomy
Purpose		
Diagnostic	Surgical exploration for diagnostic purpose	Exploratory laparotomy, breast tissue biopsy
Ablative	Removal of diseased organ	Amputation, cholecystectomy
Palliative	Performed to reduce the intensity of symptoms	Wound debridement
Reconstructive	Restores function and appearance of diseased tissue	Scar removal/revision
Constructive	Restores the damage caused due to congenital anomaly	Cleft lip, cleft palate, atrioseptal defect closure
Cosmetic	Performed for aesthetic reason	Rhinoplasty for nose repair, squint correction
Transplant	Removal of tissue or organ from a brain of dead person's body for transplanting into other's body	Kidney, liver transplant

PREOPERATIVE PERIOD

Individuals respond differently to surgical intervention. Therefore each client requires individualized nursing care planning. Patient enters the health care institution in a variety of ways ranging from a preplanned elective intervention to the emergency surgery. It is the nurse's responsibility to carry out a thorough physical assessment and teaching for her client to ensure a flawless promotion to the preoperative phase.

PREOPERATIVE ASSESSMENT

Assessment of the surgical patient helps to establish a normal baseline for the client and cautions you to meet any special needs and potential intraoperative and postoperative complications. (**Refer chapter 4 for physical examination and nursing health history.)**

Preoperative Teaching Concepts

A perioperative teaching program helps to provide the essential means to assure quality and continuity of care during the perioperative period. The term perioperative encompasses all the three phases of surgical intervention, the preoperative phase, intraoperative phase and the postoperative phase.

An effective preoperative teaching program includes input from all members of the surgical team including the perioperative nurses. A comprehensive preoperative teaching program should include the following items:

- Information regarding the sequence of events.
- Dietary restrictions.
- Preoperative part preparation.
- Preoperative medication.
- Postoperative activities—limitation, pain management.
- Family orientation—location of surgical, waiting lounge.
- Follow up visits.

Planning Perioperative Patient Care

Based on the assessment you have made, the planning, and goal-setting phase, patient care begins. This stage consists of three components:

1. Individual needs of the patient:
   - Transportation needs.
   - Emotional support.
   - Special procedures like inserting Foley's catheter, positional aids, or part preparation.
2. Possible complications:
   - Based on medical condition or diagnosis.
   - Laboratory data, nurse's notes, anesthesia evaluation.
   - Equipment and supplies anticipation.
3. Activities to be performed:
   - Based on assessment needs.
   - Patient oriented needs.
   - Specialty equipment like microscope, endoscope, monitoring devices.
   - Surgical team needs.

Admission before Surgery

When patient arrives in the ward for presurgical admission, he/she is informed about the time of admission and required fasting time.

Observation

The first task to ascertain the fitness for surgery is to record a set of baseline observation about temperature, pulse and respiration (TPR), and blood pressure (BP). Baseline observations are needed before the anesthetist reviews the patient. He needs to be informed of any untoward observations such as pyrexia, hypertension, arrhythmias, urinary tract infection (UTI) which might necessitate cancellation of the operation until the patient is well.

Weight

The patient's weight is important for drug calculation and administration. Anesthetic agents and analgesics are determined on a dose for weight (mg per kg) ratio.

Surgical History

The patient's surgical history is important to ascertain any previous complications with anesthetics or postoperative complications. History of any reaction to anesthetic agent, pacemaker insertion, any other prosthetic device, anticoagulant therapy are an important consideration during any surgery.

Medical History

The patient's medical history may determine risk factors, and if possible, should include a family health history. Frequently encountered conditions include diabetes, coronary heart disease, and hypertension.

Medications

For any medication, it is important to ascertain if the patient has any known allergies and if so, they must be clearly recorded on a medication sheet and patient's chart. All medications should be recorded including over the counter drugs. If possible, patient's compliance with medication should be recorded.

Preoperative Anesthetic Assessment

Before any operation, the anesthetist assesses the patient's medical suitability to undergo anesthesia. This is conducted in outpatient department (OPD) clinic, where the patient is seen, assessed and their anesthesia is discussed before hospitalization. The preanesthesia assessment includes information about patient's current state of health. Patient is asked about any cardiac, renal, hepatic, endocrine, respiratory or central nervous system symptoms or disease. History of any drug allergies, previous anesthesia, familial disease, drug, alcohol is questioned. Patient's airway, heart, lung and relevant tests are checked. All of these answers are evaluated as they guide the anesthetist in deciding the most appropriate type of anesthesia.

Preparation for Theater

The information obtained during the preoperative assessment, should be conveyed to the individual, responsible to prepare and transport the patient to operation room.

The admission begins with an introduction by the surgical preparatory unit nurse and a series of questions to verify data on the chart, and ends when the patient has been cleared by area personnel and shifted to operation room.

The operation room (OR) policy should have the following elements:

- Verification of patient's identification: Verbally, and by checking ID bracelet.
- Verification of completion of appropriate forms: History and physical examination, results of diagnostic studies, consent forms, preoperative assessment.
- Review of related nursing procedures performed: Nurse's notes, vital signs, allergies, diabetic chart.
- Verification of physician's orders: Elimination, medication, IV therapy, NPO status.
- Safety and comfort measures needed during the perioperative period: Removal of prosthesis, dentures and so on.
- Patient's response to preoperative medication: Physiological monitoring, pain control.

Nursing Activities

Identification and Verification

Proper patient identification includes verification of the patient, surgeon, surgical procedure and type of anesthesia.

Review of Record

Patient's record includes admission sheet, allergies, results of laboratory tests, history and physical examination, preoperative medication, specific preoperative orders of the surgeon or anesthetist.

Laboratory Data

Certain laboratory values are significant to the success of proposed surgical procedure. The nurse should review these findings and report any deviations to the appropriate person. See Table 6.2 for common preoperative laboratory tests.

Fasting

For any prebooked elective surgery, it is essential to fast before a general anesthesia. If the patient has not fasted, there is a risk of vomiting and aspiration. Within a fasting time, any oral premedication is given with a minimal amount of water (20–30 mL).

Skin Preparation

A preoperative shower with an antimicrobial skin wash is an important way of reducing a surgical site infection. Jewellery must be removed, as any metal in contact with the patient's skin can cause burns from the diathermy current. Dentures must be removed as they can dislodge during the anesthetic intubation.

Reception in Operation Room

As soon as the patient is called in the OR, he is shifted to the stretcher taking care not to injure him, cover the patient with appropriate linen and elevate the side rails. The medical record accompanies the client in the OR.

Informed Consent

Informed consent is the patient's voluntary agreement to undergo proposed procedure or treatment after receiving the following information in an understandable language by the attending physician.

Table 6.2: Common Preoperative Laboratory Investigations

Test	*Normal Range*
Hemoglobin (Hb)	Male 12–18 g/dL
	Female 10–14 g/dL
Prothrombin time (PT)	11–15 sec
Partial thromboplastin time, activated (aPTT)	24–34 sec
Hematocrit	35–47%
White blood cell count	4000–11000 cells/mL
Differential count	Segmented neutrophils 50–60%
	Eosinophils 1–4%
	Basophils 0.5–1%
	Lymphocytes 20–40%
	Monocytes 2–6%
Erythrocyte Sedimentation Rate (ESR)	41–54%
Sodium (Na^+)	136–146 mEq/L
Potassium (K^+)	3.5–5.0 mEq/L
Chloride (Cl^-)	98–108 mEq/L
Calcium (Ca^{++})	8.6–10 mEq/L
Glucose	
• Fasting	60–100 mg/dL
• Postprandial	80–120 mg/dL

- Details of the procedure.
- The underlying human pathology.
- Details of the health personnel performing the procedure.

- Proper explanation of the risk and complications involved for any disfigurement, or death and the magnitude of occurrence.
- Explanation of the patient's bill of rights, as he has full right to refuse or accept the treatment and that the consent can be withdrawn.

Informed consent safeguards the patient, physician and the health care institution. This form is a legal document. Though the responsibility to obtain the consent lays with the physician, the nurse may sign as a witness, signifying that the patient was alert, aware and conscious of the act.

PREOPERATIVE CHECKLIST

Diagnosis:

Procedure:

Date of procedure:

Yes	No	N/A	Initial	
				Height ________ Weight ______
				Preoperative orders written If 'NO', Dr ______________ notified at __________ date/time
				Consent completed
				Allergies labeled on chart
				Vital signs T ______ P ________ R ________ BP ________ Isolation label on chart
				Lab investigation placed in chart
				Urine analysis results placed in chart
				CXR with report placed in chart
				ECG report placed in chart
				Intake-output sheet placed in chart
				Medication administration sheet placed in chart
				Any special forms placed in chart
				Patient identification band in place and legible
				Bathing done and hair tied up
				OT dress worn
				Nail polish, jewellery removed Prosthesis _____ lens, dentures, hearing aid removed
				NPO since ____________am/pm
				Voided/catheterized
				Preoperative medication given
				Time ______________
				Preoperative antibiotic given
				Remarks
				Patient transported to OT on ______________
				Transportation time ______________
				Attending nurse ________________

INTRAOPERATIVE PERIOD

The intraoperative phase begins with admission of the patient to the operation room, and ends with the transfer to the designated postanesthesia area.

Members of the Surgical Team

Because of the complexity of the intraoperative environment, members of the surgical team must act as a single coordinated unit. The surgeon, surgical assistant, anesthesiologist, circulating nurse, scrub nurse, operation room technician constitutes the surgical team.

Circulating nurse is a highly experienced registered nurse responsible for managing patient care activities before, during and after the surgical procedure. Some of the activities performed by the circulating nurse are:

- Assisting and preparing the OR.
- Supervising the transportation, moving and lifting of the patient.
- Positioning the patient for surgery.
- Conducting and maintaining accurate records.
- Dispensing supplies and medications to the surgical field.
- Scrub nurse is involved in technical skills, manual dexterity and in-depth knowledge of the anatomical and mechanical aspects of particular surgery.

Transporting, Moving and Lifting the Patient

Once the OR is prepared for the procedure, the patient is transported to the designated room. Patient safety is given the primary importance while shifting. Transport the patient only after the preadmission procedure is completed. When the patient is finally on operation table the nurse applies the safety strap with brief explanation and remains with him as anesthetist prepares for induction.

Positioning the Surgical Patient

Patient positioning is a facet of patient care management that is as important to the surgical outcome as adequate preoperative preparation and safe administration of anesthesia.

The commonly used positions for most surgical procedures:

- Supine
- Prone
- Trendelenberg
- Reverse Trendelenberg
- Lithotomy
- Sitting (modified Fowler)
- Lateral recumbent.

Aseptic Practice

Asepsis refers to the condition of being free from disease causing organism. The overall goal in asepsis is to minimize contamination of the wound. The Association of Operating Room Nurses (AORN) has developed seven recommended practices for aseptic technique. AORN's guidelines are:

- Wearing sterile gowns and gloves.
- Use of sterile drapes.
- Sterility of items introduced into the sterile field.
- Maintenance of sterility and integrity of items within the sterile field.
- Monitoring and maintaining the sterile field.
- Traffic patterns in the sterile field.
- Policies and procedures for basic aseptic technique.

Introduction of Anesthesia

Nature of the operative procedure and the patient's physical condition influences the type of anesthesia to be administered. A brief overview of various types of anesthesia is given below:

- **General anesthesia:** General anesthesia involves the administration of drugs by inhalation, intravenous, rectal or oral route to produce central nervous system depression. General anesthesia results in overall loss of sensation, consciousness, relaxed skeletal muscles and depressed reflexes.
- **Regional anesthesia:** Regional anesthesia involves the injection of anesthetic agent in or around the operative site, blocking the transmission of sensory stimuli to central nervous system receptors. The patient receiving regional anesthesia remains fully conscious and awake, but loses sensation in specific area. Regional anesthesia is given through (a) major nerve blocks, (b) subarachnoid (spinal), (c) caudal and/or epidural blocks.
  - **Nerve blocks:** Nerve blocks involve injecting a local anesthetic around a nerve trunk supplying the area of surgery.
  - **Spinal anesthesia:** Spinal anesthesia is accomplished by injecting a local anesthetic into the subarachnoid space through a lumbar puncture, resulting in sensory, motor and autonomic blockage.
  - **Caudal and epidural anesthesia:** Caudal anesthesia is the injection of local anesthetic into epidural space through the caudal canal in the sacrum. Epidural anesthesia involves injecting the drug through the intervertebral spaces, usually in the lumbar region.
- **Topical and local anesthesia:** Topical anesthesia is used on mucus membranes, open skin surfaces and wounds. Xylocaine 10% is the most commonly used agent. Local anesthesia is the injection of an anesthetic agent like xylocaine to a specific area of body.
- **Conscious sedation/analgesia:** Conscious sedation/analgesia is used for procedures where simply a decreased level of consciousness is desired. The patient maintains cardiorespiratory function and can respond to verbal commands. Advantages of IV conscious sedation

are diminished anxiety, adequate sedation, increased pain threshold, amnesia and enhanced patient cooperation.

Draping

Drapes are used to maintain a sterile field around the operative site. The only area left exposed is the incision site.

Documenting

Throughout surgery, the perioperative nurse is responsible to document the ongoing patient assessment, item counts, monitoring data, positioning, medications, dressings and drains so forth on the intraoperative record.

Transferring to the postanesthesia care unit (PACU): After the operation, the patient is carefully shifted from operation table to the stretcher. The patient is then transported to the PACU with complete reporting of preoperative and intraoperative assessments and interventions to the PACU nurse, to ensure continuity of care.

POSTOPERATIVE PERIOD

The postoperative phase of the perioperative period begins with the transfer of the patient to designated postanesthesia area and ends with the resolution of the surgical experience. Before the transfer is accomplished, the following activities should be completed by perioperative nurse.

- Intraoperative documentation is completed and reviewed for accuracy.
- Proper identification, labeling and placing of specimen in appropriate containers.
- Arrangement for any special equipment as requested for postanesthesia care.
- Patient is moved to a recovery bed and transported to the PACU.
- Verbal/written report is given to the appropriate PACU nurse.

Primary Objectives of Postanesthesia Nursing Care

There are four primary objective of nursing care in PACU:

1. Recognize the major potential problems associated with performed surgical procedure, and the appropriate corresponding actions.
2. Identify and demonstrate the general procedures routinely carried out in the PACU area.
3. Maintain accurate documentation of the patient's progress during the recovery phase.
4. Recognize and use the criteria for discharging a patient from the PACU, to the subsequent area of patient care.

Management of Patient Care in PACU

Initial Assessment Activities

The primary goal of immediate postanesthesia nursing care is the safe recovery and arousal of patient from the effects of anesthesia. The initial assessment of the patient should include the following areas:

- Vital signs:
  - Respiratory status
  - Circulatory status
  - Pulse
  - Temperature
  - Oxygen saturation level
- Color and condition of skin and mucus membranes
- Hemodynamic values
- Patient position
- Type and patency of drainage tubes and catheters
- Condition of dressings (with attention to amount and type of drainage)
- Activity status, extremity movement
- Level of consciousness, response to stimuli
- Level of comfort/safety
  - Pain
  - Status of protective reflexes
- IV therapy; patency of catheters

Nursing Diagnosis Statements

Based on assessment and observation, nurse is in position to identify the nursing diagnoses that are applied to her client. These diagnoses give way to progressive patient care in PACU and surgical nursing unit.

Nursing diagnoses for postoperative client
Airway clearance: ineffective
Anxiety
Activity intolerance
Body image disturbance
Breathing pattern: ineffective
Communication: impaired verbal
Constipation: risk for
Fluid volume: risk for deficient
Infection: risk for
Mobility: impaired physical
Nausea
Nutrition imbalance: less than body needs
Pain acute
Sleep pattern: disturbed
Tissue perfusion: ineffective
Urinary elimination: impaired
Ventilation: impaired spontaneous

Planning

The use of standardized care plans for the postanesthesia area provides continuity of patient care, since more than one recovery nurse is involved in patient care during the recovery phase. The care plan should incorporate all aspects of postanesthesia care and should be modified according to the needs of individual patients.

Objectives

While recovering in the PACU, goals of care include returning back to normal physiological parameters without complications and maintaining physical and psychological comfort. The patient should also be conscious and oriented to PACU set up, with the ability to move four extremities and to verbalize pain relief and reduced anxiety. When the client is shifted to surgical nursing unit, goals are long-term in nature. Wound healing, restoring health status, pain relief are few examples.

Setting priorities

In PACU, patient priorities gyrate around physiological needs. The nurse here determines the patient progress, and set priorities on changing needs to prevent any untoward complications. Even in the surgical nursing unit to maintain physical status, it is important to be cautious for developing complications. If the patient's pain is properly managed, ambulation begins early, he will have a better sense of well-being.

Continuity of care

Continuous care management depends on good communication among the members of surgical team. Nurse in each area must be able to share clear and accurate information about the client status, to the next level nurse who assumes responsibility for the client.

Implementation

Analytical thinking is of great importance in the postoperative period, because the nurse considers the interrelationship of all body systems. The risk of postoperative complications is constantly there if a thorough care is not given and the client is not involved in his care. Few nursing interventions for a smooth patient care are:

Respiration

- Position the client on one side with neck little extended and face little downward.
- Suction the airway and oral cavity for mucus secretions as needed.
- Initiate deep breathing and coughing exercise as early as possible.
- Administer oxygen as ordered, but monitor oxygen saturation with pulse oximeter.

Circulation

- Check blood pressure and heart rate.
- Encourage to perform leg exercises at least every hour unless contraindicated.
- Encourage early ambulation.
- Promote adequate fluid intake orally or intravenously.

Thermoregulation: Provide warm blankets or warming devices.

Fluid and electrolyte balance

- Administer IV fluids as ordered.
- Maintain the patency of IV line.
- Regulate the rate of infusion as ordered. An infusion pump may be required for a seriously ill client.

Neurological functions

- Address the client by name in a soft tone to test his level of response.
- Orient the client to his new environment.

Genitourinary functions

- Assist the client to assume normal position for voiding.
- Ask for the need to void when a catheter is not in place.
- Assess for bladder distension, as difficulty in voiding may require an indwelling catheter.
- Monitor intake and output charting.

Remember: If the output is less than 30 mL/hr the client might be experiencing acute renal failure and immediate notification of the surgeon is imperative.

Gastrointestinal functions

- Maintain a gradual progression in dietary intake.
- Encourage ambulation and exercise.
- Maintain an adequate fluid intake.
- Administer fiber supplements, stool softeners, enema or rectal suppositories as prescribed.
- Provide a thorough oral hygiene.
- Stimulate appetite by keeping away any source of noxious odors and small sized meals.

Comfort

- Administer pain medications as and when prescribed.
- Comfortable positions also reduce stress to an extent.

Wound healing

- Leave surgical dressings in place to decrease the risk of infection.
- Notify the surgeon for excessive bleeding.
- Check the patency of surgical drains to prevent accumulation of secretions.
- Observe the wound for any signs of infection (redness, heat, edema, odor, purulent drainage).

Maintaining self-concept

- Provide privacy during procedures or any exposure.
- Maintain hygiene of your patient.
- Maintain pleasant environment.
- Provide opportunity to discuss his feeling about appearance and self-concept.

Evaluation and Discharge

Before discharge the attending anesthesia practitioner assesses the patient's readiness to leave the unit. Postanesthesia discharge criteria is as follows:

- Patient maintains a clear airway
- Vital signs are stable
- Protective reflexes are active
- Patient is conscious and oriented
- Adequate intake and output (urinary output of 30 mL/hr)
- Afebrile
- Dressings are dry and intact with no overt drainage

To provide continuity of care a detailed verbal report of patient's status is given to the next nurse responsible for continuing postoperative management of this patient. Once the client is shifted to surgical nursing unit, it is important to evaluate the effectiveness of care on the basis of expected outcomes. Nurse's evaluation is an ongoing technique that occurs over several days. It is significant to evaluate the patient's clinical progress by observing his degree of participation in postoperative activities such as self-care activities, exercises, ambulation.

Even a telephonic call in the first 24 hours of his hospital discharge to his home helps the nurse to assess home-care outcomes. This not only allows you to evaluate the progress of recovery but also answer any questions the client may have.

7 Nursing Pharmacology

OBJECTIVES

After completion of this chapter, students will be able to:

- Discuss drug legislation in India.
- Comprehend the role of a nurse in drug administration.
- Develop skills in drug administration to patients.
- Identify the effects of variety of drugs used in therapeutics.
- Identify the drug classification.
- Identify the routes of administration of drugs.
- Discuss the types of drugs and their actions.
- Calculate drug dosages, using various formulas and system of measurement.
- Explain various safety factors involved in drug administration.

A drug or medication is any substance that modifies body physiology when consumed in the body. Therefore, **pharmacology** may be defined as the study of drugs. This includes their origin, chemical structure, preparation, administration, actions, metabolism and excretion. Medication or drug is a chemical substance used in diagnostic, therapeutic and preventive aspects of a disease.

DRUG LEGISLATION RELATED TO TOBACCO AND DRUGS

The Drug and Cosmetics Act, 1940 (Amended in 1964, 1983) is an Act to regulate the import, manufacture, distribution and sale of drugs and cosmetics. It extends to the whole of India.

The Narcotic Drugs and Psychotropic Substances Act, 1985

This Act deals with narcotic drugs, psychotropic substance (Cannabis, opium, poppy straw, cola) and property derived from or used in illicit traffic in narcotic drugs and psychotropic substances and to implement the provisions of the international conventions on narcotic drugs and psychotropic substances. It extends to the whole of India.

Delhi Antismoking and Nonsmoker's Health Protection Act, 1996

According to this Act, smoking is prohibited in public places so that nonsmokers can be protected from exposure to tobacco smoke.

USE OF DRUGS

In the treatment of any client, a therapeutic plan must be designed to decide the realistic objectives of treatment. This plan includes the use of drugs, but certain factors should be kept in mind:

- Is the drug appropriate for the disorder and the client being treated?
- What has been the client's response to the drug in the past? A complete drug history is essential.
- Does the patient understand the implications of treatment?
- Has the correct therapy been chosen?

TYPES OF DRUGS AND THEIR MODE OF ACTION

- *General anesthetics* depress cerebral function, induce unconsciousness and prevent all sensation.
- *Local anesthetics* interfere with the function of a nerve or nerve ending and prevent all sensation from a localized areas without loss of consciousness.

- *Analgesics* relieve pain without interfering with consciousness.
- *Anthelmintics* kills or aids the removal of worms from the intestines.
- *Antiepileptics* prevent fits.
- *Antipyretics* reduce body temperature when it is raised above normal
- *Antibiotics* are prepared from living organism and kill or prevent multiplication of bacteria in the body.
- *Aperients* loosen the bowels.
- *Carminatives* promote belching.
- *Chemotherapeutic* agents are prepared synthetically to kill or prevent the multiplication of bacteria within the body.
- *Contraceptives* prevent conception.
- *Cytotoxic* agents are drugs which damage or kill malignant cells and are used in treating cancers.
- *Diaphoretics* induce sweating.
- *Disinfectants* kill bacteria.
- *Diuretics* increase the secretion of urine.
- *Emetics* produce vomiting.
- *Expectorants* make the bronchial secretions more liquid and therefore more easily expelled.
- *Hypnotics* produce sleep.
- *Hypotensive* drugs lower blood pressure.
- *Mydriatics* dilate the pupil.
- *Myotics* constrict the pupil.
- *Neuroleptics* are anti-psychotic drugs.
- *Opioids* have a similar action to opium.
- *Prodrug* is substance which is inactive, but is converted into an active drug in the body.
- *Sedatives* soothe, but may also cause drowsiness.
- *Styptics* stop local bleeding.
- *Tonics* are said to restore general well-being, but are of doubtful value.
- *Tranquilizers* promote mental relaxation without drowsiness.

DRUG ADMINISTRATION

In hospital the custody and administration of drugs is the responsibility of the ward sister/charge nurse, who may delegate this role according to the employing authority's policy. Terminology referring to drug administration and the various routes of administering a medication are given in Tables 7.1 and 7.2 respectively.

Table 7.1: Terminology referring to drug administration.

a.c.	Before meals
Ad lib	As much as required
b.d.s.	Twice daily
b.i.d.	Twice daily
Gutt	Drops
i.m.	Intramuscular
inj.	Injection
I.U.	International units
I.V.	Intravenous
o.h.	Every hour
o.m.	Every morning
o.n.	Every night
p.c.	After meals
p.o.	Orally
p.r.	Per rectum
P.V.	Per vagina
q.d.s.	Four times daily
q.i.d.	Four times daily
rep.	Repeat
s.o.s.	If necessary
Stat	At once
t.d.s.	Three times daily
t.i.d.	Three times daily

Table 7.2: Routes of administration

Oral route	By swallowing
Enteral route	Through an enteral tube
Sublingual	Placing a drug under the tongue
Buccal	Placing a drug between cheek and gum
Parenteral route	By injecting the drug into
Subcutaneous	Subcutaneous tissue
Intramuscular	Muscular tissue
Intradermal	Dermis
Intravenous	Vein
Intra-arterial	Artery
Intracardial	Heart
Intraspinal	Spinal canal
Introsseous	Bone tissue
Intrathecal	Subarachnoid space
Topical route	By inserting the medication into
Vaginal	Vagina

Contd...

Contd...

Rectal	Rectum
Inunction	Rubbing over the skin
Instillation	Drug infused in contact with mucous membrane
Irrigation	Flushing of mucous membrane with drug solution
Respiratory route	By inhaling the drug

NURSING RESPONSIBILITIES IN DRUG ADMINISTRATION

The nurse is responsible for interpreting the prescription accurately, recording that the drug has been given and observing the patient's response. Observations shall be made for therapeutic and adverse effects.

Whichever approach is taken safely is prime concern while preparing and implementing drug administration.

The **six rights** that ensure accuracy when administering medications are:

1. Right medication
2. Right patient
3. Right dose
4. Right route
5. Right time
6. Right documentation

The label on the drug container should be checked exactly ***three times*** during its preparation. **First** it should be checked while reaching for the container, **second** immediately before opening the medication, **third** when replacing the container to the medication trolley or shelf or before giving the unit dose medication to the patient.

Ask the attending physician for any doubt or confusion.

MEDICATION ORDERS

Drug administration shall not be performed without prescribed orders from a treating physician. Every health care institution has a fixed policy specifying the way the physician writes an order. Though a nurse may receive an order in writing, in verbal or telephonically, but safe practice commands that she follows only the written orders.

Types of Orders

- *Written orders:* Written orders are the ones that a physician writes on a standard physician/medication order sheet.
- *Verbal orders:* Verbal orders are received in the presence of attending physician. These are generally given in emergency situations, however the physician signs them later. Nurses should generally refrain from following verbal orders and ask the physician to do so in written format.
- *Telephonic orders:* Telephonic orders are received in telephone when a nurse reports some change in patient's condition or upon the arrival of some investigation report.

Components of Medication Order

- Patient's name.
- Date and time of writing an order.
- Medication name.
- Dosage of the drug.
- Route of administration.
- Frequency of administration.
- Physician signature.

Common Medication Error

Drug administration requires all carefulness to prevent occurrence of any untoward incidence. Common medication errors that might occur while administering are:

- Inappropriate prescription in term of incorrect dose, route, time.
- Extra, omitted and incorrect doses.
- Administering medication to wrong patient, e.g. similar name confusion.
- Drug administration by incorrect route.
- Delay in recording the drug administration can result in repetition of the drug.
- Inadequate knowledge of dosage calculations formulae.

SAFETY FACTORS IN PREVENTING MEDICATION ERRORS

- Do not leave the drug trolley unattended.
- Do not give drug from memory; a prescription sheet must always be used.
- Do not give a drug from a container which is not correctly labeled.
- Do not give a drug prepared by someone else.
- Do not replace the unused dose to a stock bottle.
- Unused drugs should be returned back to pharmacy where they are checked and used for another patient.
- Follow six rights to prevent error.
- Carry out three checks carefully
- Get the calculation checked by a fellow nurse while preparing medication.

PATIENTS EDUCATION AND COMPLIANCE TO THERAPEUTIC REGIMEN

In order to comply an understanding and acceptance of the treatment is vital, failure to do so may be unintentional due to lapse of memory, or deliberate, when dosage may be altered by the patient. Patient education is the responsibility of the physician, pharmacist and nurse, however the quantum of the information must be tailored to the individual needs but must include the following:

- The name and purpose of the drug stressing its positive effects.
- Frequency and timing of administration, according to home routine, including advice about 'as required' medications.
- Method of administration with explanation where special equipment is required for routes other than oral,
- The importance of not stopping or starting drugs without advice and where to obtain that advice.
- Adverse effects to be reported.
- How to obtain further supplies and safely dispose of unwanted drugs.

DOSAGE CALCULATION

Patients may be prescribed doses of a drug which are not precisely equivalent to a single tablet, ampoule or 5 mL spoonful. Therefore, it is essential to calculate the quantity of drugs preparation which will contain the dose prescribed as this is a common source of error in drug administration.

Dosage calculation is a worry to nurses (and others). The following list of formulae will help to overcome the fear of wrong dosage calculation.

1. **Parenteral dosage**

$$\frac{\text{Dose prescribed}}{\text{Dose available}} \times \text{quantity in hand (mL = volume to be given)}$$

2. **Intravenous fluid drop rate**

$$\frac{\text{Total volume to be infused}}{\text{Time in minutes}} \times \text{drop factor} = \text{drop rate/min}$$

3. **Insulin dose**

$$\frac{\text{What we want}}{\text{What we have}} \times \text{No. of divisions on the syringe}$$

4. **Concentration**

$$\frac{\text{Dosage of drug (in mg)}}{\text{Volume to be infused}} \times 1000$$

Pediatric formulae

5. **Fried's form (For infants)**

$$\frac{\text{Age in months}}{\text{150 months}} \times \text{Average adult dose}$$

6. **Young's rule (For children up to 12 years old)**

$$\frac{\text{Child's age in years}}{\text{Child's age in years + 12}} \times \text{Average adult dose}$$

7. **Clark's rule**

$$\frac{\text{Weight in pounds}}{\text{150 pounds}} \times \text{Average adult dose}$$

8. **Body surface area rule**

$$\frac{\text{Body surface area in sq m}}{1.73} \times \text{Average adult dose}$$

SYSTEM OF MEASUREMENT

Three basic systems of drug calculation are: (i) the metric system, (ii) the apothecary system and (iii) the household system. Nurse needs to gain proficiency in calculating and converting the dosage from one system to another.

Metric System

The metric system is the most commonly practiced system. The basic units of metric system are meter (length), liter (volume) and gram (weight).

Weight

1 g = 1000 mg
1 kg = 1000 g
0.001 g = 1 mg
0.001 kg = 1 g
1 mg = 1000 μg

Volume

1 L = 1000 mL
1 mL = 1 cubic centimeter
0.001 L = 1 mL

Length

1 meter = 100 cm
1 cm = 10 mm
1 mm = 0.1 cm

Apothecary System

Apothecary system is not used frequently. The units of weight is grain, the unit of volume is minim.

Weight

60 grain = 1 dram
8 drain = 1 ounce

Volume

60 minims = 1 fluid dram (fl dr)
8 fl dr = 1 fluid ounce (oz)
16 fl oz = 1 pint (1 pt)
2 pt = 1 quart (qt)

Household System

This system is practiced in home care setting

5 mL = 1 teaspoon (tsp)
15 mL = 1 tablespoon (Tbsp)
180 mL = 1 cupful
240 mL = 1 glassful

8 Operation Theater Nursing

OBJECTIVES

After completion of this chapter, students will be able to:

- Identify the principles of medical-surgical asepsis.
- Create safe environment for surgical patients.
- Develop skills in administering personalized care to OT patients.
- Develop a sense of surgical team-membership.
- Explain conditions that could result in nosocomial infections.
- Get acquainted with wide variety of instrument being used in different surgeries.
- Discuss the role of a theater nurse.
- Explain various methods of sterilization and disinfection.

SECTION I

An operation theater provides a place where surgical procedures are undertaken with maximum safety for the patient. It is a complex engineering to provide power for lighting, ventilation, working machines and meeting many more demands that are essential for the care of the patient.

ASEPSIS AND THEATER TECHNIQUE

Asepsis is the underlying principle of surgery by which microbes are denied any access to the patient.

Asepsis is defined as the absence of disease causing organisms. Asepsis has a concrete discipline of its own, all efforts aimed at keeping the patient as free from infection is known as *aseptic technique.*

There are two types of aseptic techniques which are being practiced are medical asepsis and surgical asepsis.

Medical Asepsis (Clean Technique)

Medical asepsis covers procedures used to reduce the number of microorganisms and to prevent their spread. Hand washing, barrier technique and routine environmental cleaning are few examples of medical asepsis.

Principles of Medical Asepsis

- Frequent hand washing, and before and after every procedure.
- Clean from more cleaner to less cleaner area.
- Follow biomedical waste segregation.
- Follow barrier technique as prescribed by your hospital.
- Follow damp dusting technique to prevent spreading of dust and organisms.

Surgical Asepsis

Surgical asepsis means total absence of any organism (both pathogenic and non-pathogenic) and their spores from an article, area or environment. Surgical asepsis includes procedures like operations, care of wound, urinary catheterization, etc.

Principles of Surgical Asepsis

- A sterile object remains sterile only when touched by another sterile object.
- Place a sterile object only on a sterile field.
- A sterile object or field out of visual range or an object below a waist level is contaminated.
- A sterile object or field is contaminated by capillary action when a sterile surface comes in contact with a wet contaminated surface.
- Because fluids flow towards gravity, a sterile object gets contaminated if gravity causes a contaminated fluid to flow over the object's surface.
- Edges of sterile field are contaminated.

Practical Points of Importance

1. Air consists of dust and droplet particles, which allows dissemination of airborne organisms. To minimize the bacterial count of the air following precaution should be taken:
   - Ventilation: Ideally air should be filtered, moistened and warmed or cooled at regular temperature. For air conditioned rooms windows should be always closed.
   - Speech should be minimal and mask worn for elimination of droplets.
   - Bodily movements should be gentle and unhurried.
   - Cleaning procedures should be completed 1 or 2 hours prior to the use of theater with a disinfectant.
2. Many objects cannot be sterilized. These include patient's skin, throat, nose and mouth of the staff.
3. The operating table and floor get contaminated from infected material during the operation.
4. Recontamination of sterile objects can occur due to inefficient sterilization, inefficient air conditioning and poor handling of sterilized instruments and other articles.
5. Theater attire should be laundered daily.
6. No jewelery should be worn.
7. Blankets are a source of infection and should be changed after each patient.

Theater Design

Because of the significance of maintaining asepsis, OT should be designed so that they have:

- Air conditioned ventilation.
- Easily cleanable fabric.
- A one-way traffic circulation from 'clean' area to 'dirty' area.

THEATER TECHNIQUE

A theater nurse and all theater staff carefully follows all the principles and techniques to prevent any kind of infection to the patient.

Theater Dress

The nurse shall be responsible to clean her person, skin uncracked and abrasion free. Nails well trimmed and unvarnished. She must wear only the OT attire which consists of a 2-piece dress (short sleeve top and loose trousers). All hair should be well concealed under the OT cap. Special footwear which is worn only in OT premises. Always wear a mask covering the nose and mouth while operation is in progress or while preparing the theater.

Theater Bedding

No ward linen should be allowed in the theater as they are a source of infection. Change the top linen while receiving the patient in the operation theater.

Theater Nurse

Whilst the operation is going on, two kinds of nurses are involved based on their role they play at this time. These are a scrub nurse and the circulating nurse.

Scrub Nurse

A scrub nurse is the one who assists the surgeon in performing the operation. It is the scrub nurse who is responsible for the instruments. She does a surgical hand scrub for 5 minutes using an antiseptic solution/soap, and dons an OT sterile attire (sterile gown, gloves) which is pulled on and tied back by the circulating nurse.

Once scrubbed, nurse now handles only the sterilized material. If inadvertently touches something that is non-sterile she must change her gown and gloves. She supervises the instruments, prepares ligatures and sutures and keeps the surgeon supplied with swabs, tubes or anything needed during the operation.

It is the duty of the scrub nurse at the end of operation, to check and count all the instruments and materials used.

Circulatory Nurse

A circulatory nurse is a great assistance to the scrub nurse, as she assembles all the articles required during the operation. She is responsible for supplying all additional equipment for the surgical team and for assisting in swab check procedure. It is also the duty of circulatory nurse to receive the specimen obtained from surgery and send it for bacteriological or histological examination after proper sealing and labeling so that patient's identity is unmistakable.

Septic Case—Theater Clearance

The primary aim of theater clearance is to confine the infected materials to one operating room by restricting movement of contaminated staff. Keep the quantity of equipment and materials to the minimum. Precautions should be followed from the beginning of the operation contaminated with pathogens.

- A towel/thick lint soaked in a disinfectant is placed on the floor of the theater entrance as a mat.
- Any equipment not to be used during the surgery is removed.
- Swabs and towels shall not be dropped on the floor but discarded in the plastic bag.
- Personnel involved should avoid leaving the room during the procedure.
- The circulating nurse should wear rubber gloves for swab count.
- Instruments after thorough washing should be immediately returned to CSSD and inform them that they are infected. Swabs are packed in plastic bag and sent for incineration. All staff should change into a clean clothing afterwards and theater is thoroughly cleaned with disinfectant (e.g. carbolic acid) before next use.

Accident Prevention in Operation Theater

In the operation theater patient and staff are at risk of burns or explosion injuries, these can be avoided by remembering the following:

Anesthetic explosion: When inflammable anesthetic agents are used, presence of any natal flame or spark can induce violent explosions, resulting in extensive burns and death of a patient or theater staff.

Static electricity: Static electricity is generated by two opposite (positive and negative) charges, which when separated produce and spark and hence electric current is generated, e.g. wool and nylon together builds up static current. Following precautions are important:

- All metallic apparatus should be fitted by antistatic rubber.
- Earthing of all apparatus.
- Maintaining safe humidity level of 60%.

Surgical diathermy: Surgical diathermy is a very high frequency electric current produced by diathermy machine. If the patient is lying on the operation table touching metal, he will be burnt at the point of contact if he is not earthed.

Electrical equipment: All electrical equipment in the OT should be checked regularly for faults and repaired immediately.

It is the duty of all the theater staff to make themselves well conversant with different kinds of impending injuries in the theater as the patient's life will be at risk.

STERILIZATION

Sterilization is a process of complete destruction and elimination of all types of microorganism (pathogenic and non-pathogenic) and vegetative spores.

Disinfection is a process of killing microorganisms by physical and chemical methods.

Methods of Sterilization

Broadly speaking, there are two methods of sterilization, physical methods and chemical methods.

Physical Methods

Physical methods are further classified as (a) Moist heat sterilization, (b) Dry heat sterilization, (c) Radiation method.

(a) Moist Heat Sterilization

Moist heating is the most effective method of sterilization. Moist heat is applied by boiling and autoclaving.

Boling: Water boils at 100°C. Articles are boiled at 100°C for 15–25 minutes to maintain medical asepsis. Sharp instruments like knives, scissors are never boiled for the risk of becoming blunt.

Autoclaving: Principle of steam under pressure is used for sterilization. Autoclaving is the best and most effective method of sterilizing the equipment. Temperature of 121°C (249°F), with pressure at 15 lbs/inch^2 or 1.05 kg/cm^2 for 20–30 minutes is enough to render the articles thoroughly sterile.

(b) Dry Heat Sterilization

Dry heat sterilization is used for the articles that are good conductors of heat. Dry heat is applied by hot air. A high temperature of 160°C (320°F) for 1–3 hours is applied to the equipment placed inside hot air oven. This method is used to sterilize ointments, oils, powders, LP needles, metal canula. Keep the door closed while sterilizing the equipment.

(c) Radiation Method

Radiation is a physical method of sterilization where sterilization is achieved by ultraviolet rays and gamma rays.

Ultraviolet rays or sunlight sterilization: Sunlight is a rich source of UV rays. After mechanical cleaning articles are exposed to sunlight for 6–8 hours to achieve surface sterilization. Hospital mattress, blankets, pillows are sterilized by this method.

Gamma rays sterilization: Gamma rays have high penetrating power. These are used to sterilize heat sensitive articles like syringes, IV sets, IV cannula, drugs, sutures, etc.

Chemical Methods

Disinfectants are chemical agents that are used to kill and/or prevent the growth of microorganisms.

Most chemical agents act as disinfectant and antiseptic as well, depending on the strength used, e.g. carbolic acid 1:20 is disinfectant and 1:80 is an antiseptic.

The chief varieties of disinfectants are (a) Coal tar derivatives (b) Dyes, (c) Acidic compounds (d) Heavy metals, (e) Oxidizing agents (f) Halogens, (g) Alcohols, (h) Acids, (i) Alkalies (j) Soaps and detergents.

(a) Coal Tar Derivatives

- Phenol or carbolic acid is an excellent disinfectant due to its corrosive action. 5% carbolic lotion is enough to carbolize the operation theater.
- Lysol is used to disinfect instruments, furniture, etc. Sharp instruments are soaked in pure Lysol to be sterilized. Lysol is a solution of cresol with soap.
- Savlon and Dettol are other agents which are used for cleaning of wounds, dressings, and disinfect instruments.

(b) Dyes

Gentian violet 1% is used for boiling and burning injuries. Acriflavin and Proflavin inhibits the growth of gram -ve bacteria.

(c) Acridine Compounds

Acridine compounds include flavine, euflavine, proflavin compound, which are used for dressing of wounds.

(d) Heavy Metals

Heavy metals are the compounds of mercury, silver, copper and zinc which have both bacteriostatic and bactericidal effect e.g. mercurochrome is used for skin asepsis.

(e) Oxidizing Agents

Nascent oxygen is highly destructive to bacteria compounds like potassium permanganate, hydrogen peroxide that are used for cleaning of septic wounds.

(f) Halogens

Compounds of Iodine and Chlorine are used for their rapid bactericidal action. Chlorine in gaseous form is used for disinfection of water. Calcium hypochlorite ($CaClO_2$) or bleaching powder is toxic to bacteria and 0.5 to 1% solution kills most bacteria in one to five minutes.

Iodine is another effective element of halogen family. Iodine in tincture form (alcoholic solution) is used for cuts, abrasion, and preoperative skin preparation.

(g) Alcohols

Alcohol when diluted with water becomes more germicidal. Staphylococci gets killed in 50% alcohol within an hour or two, but survive in 90% alcohol for many days, Methylated spirit is another product used for skin preparation before operative procedures.

(h) Acids

Nitric acid, hydrochloric acid, sulfuric acid are powerful acids known for their corrosive action. It is the corrosive nature of those mineral acids which limits their using, they are excessively destructive to the tissue.

(i) Alkalis

Formalin is used for preservation of tissues/specimen. Formalin gas is used for fumigation of infected rooms. Instruments are sterilized in pure formalin as it kills even spores.

(j) Soaps and Detergents

Soaps and detergents have a cleansing effects. Cinthol soap (chlorhexidine 3%) kills *meningococci* and *pneumococci* due to its chemical effects. It is also simple mechanical friction that rids hands of many bacteria after washing under running water.

SECTION II

OPERATION THEATER INSTRUMENTS

The spectrum of surgical procedure is vast and each procedure has its own instrumentation requirements. It is essential for operation theater nurse that she must be familiar with hundreds of instruments— nomenclature, usage, care and sterilization technique.

This section on surgical instruments will help all students to identify the commonly used instruments and the operations in which they are used.

Instruments differ in structure and design to fulfill specific purposes, requirements and preferences of individual surgeons. Nomenclature is not standardized as certain manufacturing companies name the instrument after its origin. However, in this section the most recognized names from the manufacturing units have been used.

The term set and instruments is significant. **Set** is a group of instruments that are used to do a certain surgery; but the term **instrument** is a single identifying unit in the set used for surgery.

The functions of the instruments are used to classify them:

1. *Cutting instruments*
2. *Grasping instruments*
3. *Clamping instruments*
4. *Exposing instruments*

CUTTING INSTRUMENTS

Cutting instruments are also referred to as sharps, because of their usable part being cutting or sharp edges. These include scalpels (knife handles with blades), scissors, osteotomes, chisels, saws, drills, curettes etc.

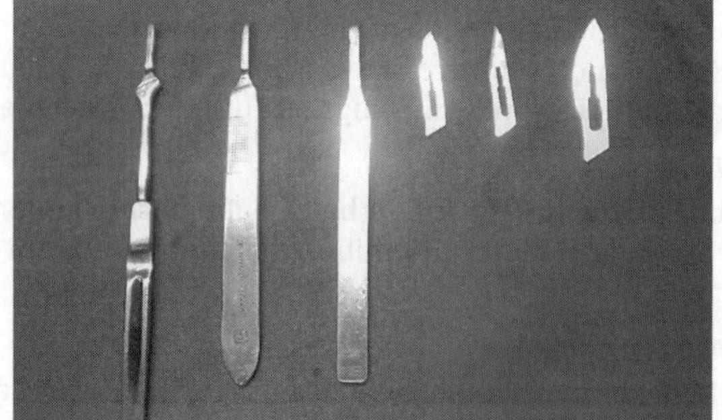

Bard parker handle (size 7, 3, 4)
Blade (size 15, 11, 23)

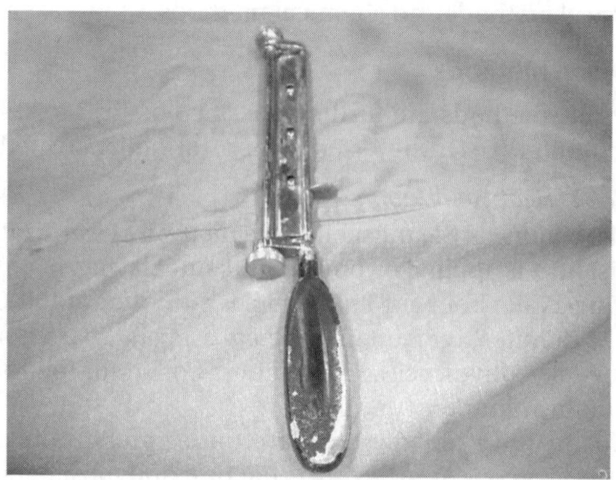

Skin grafting knife

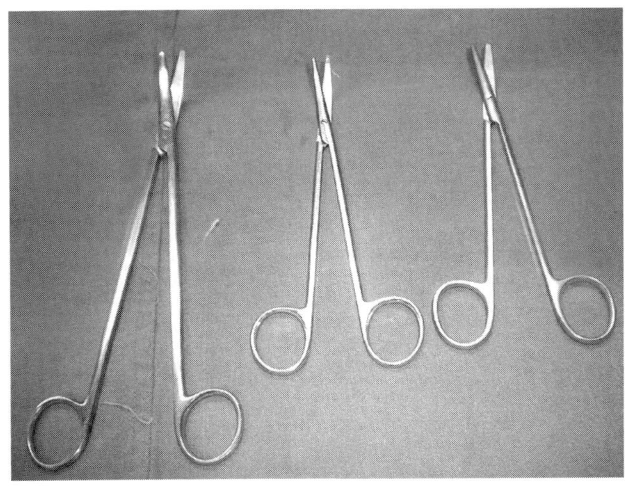

Scissors—Mayo's tissue cutting (long, medium, small)

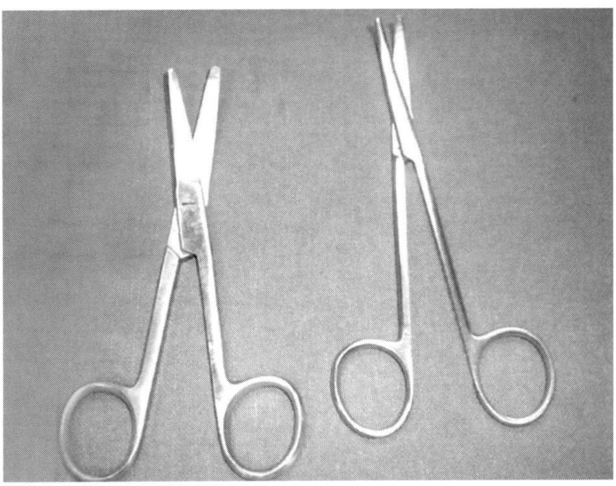

Scissors—gauze cutting

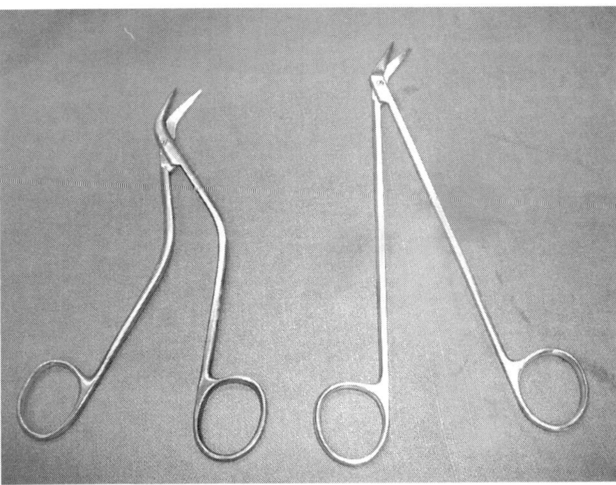

Kelly's scissors

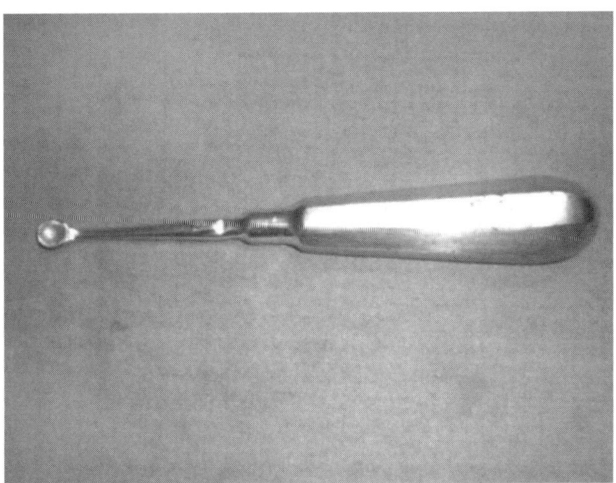

Bone curette

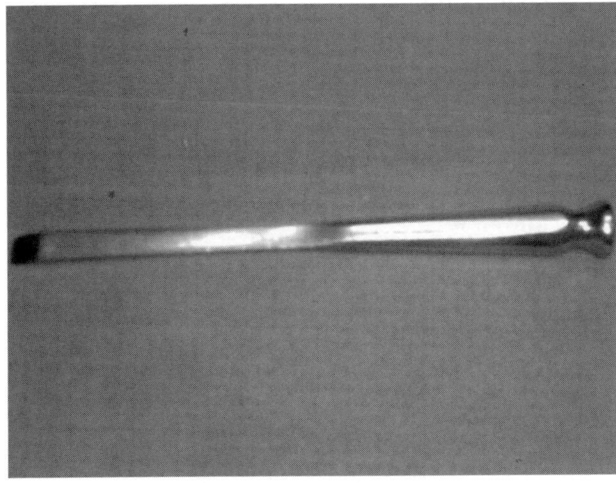

Adson laminectomy chisel

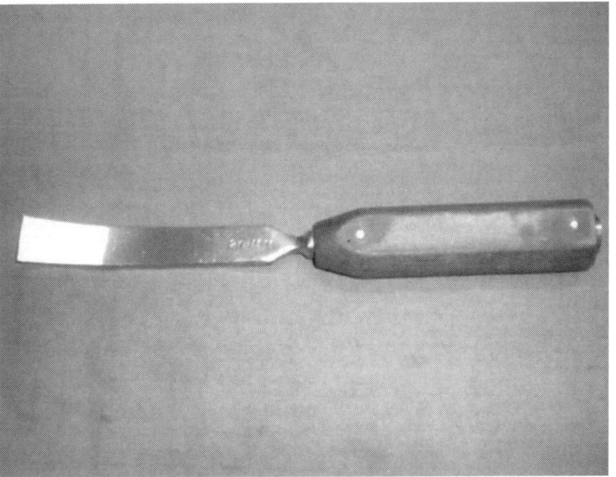

Hoke osteotome

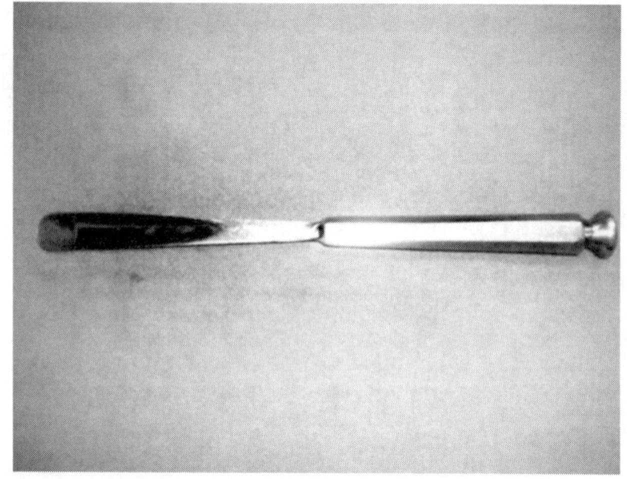

Smith-Petersen bone gouge

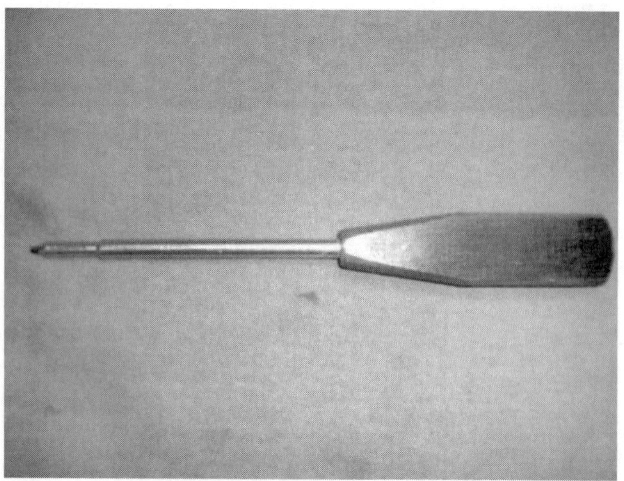

Screw driver

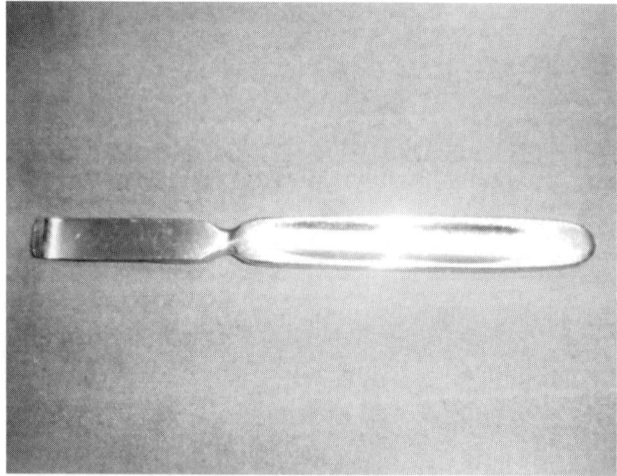

Periosteal elevator

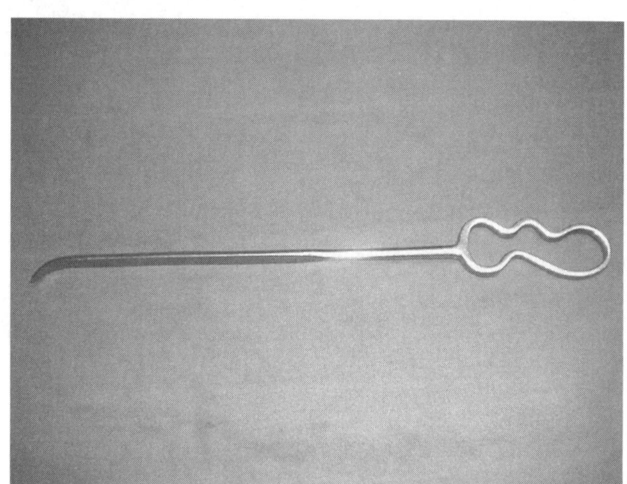

Spike

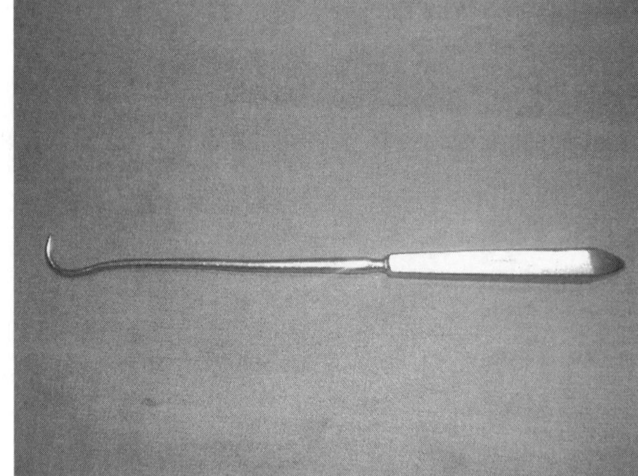

Bone hook

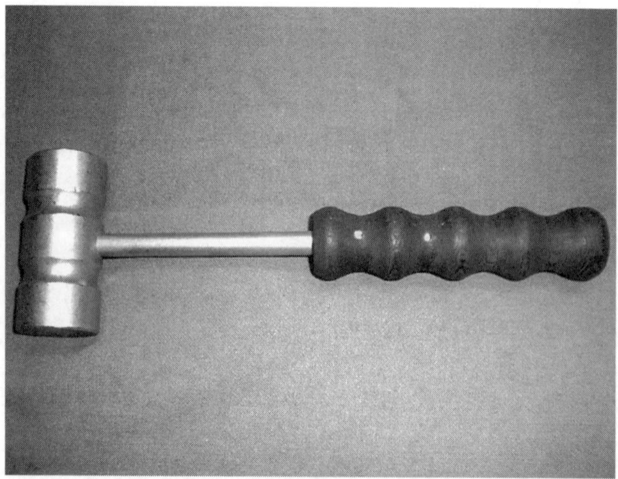

Hammer

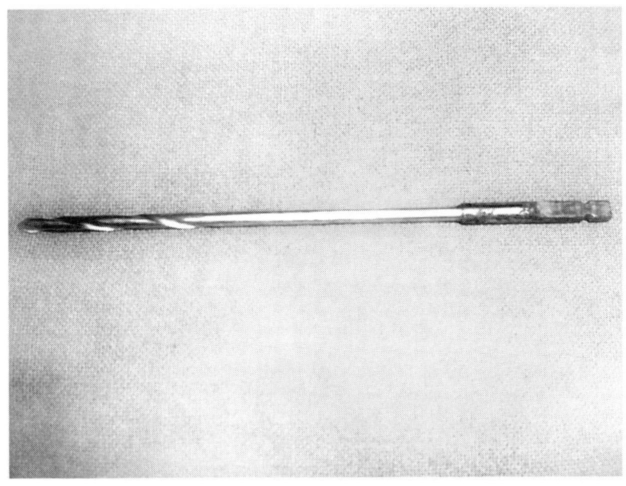

Bone drill twist

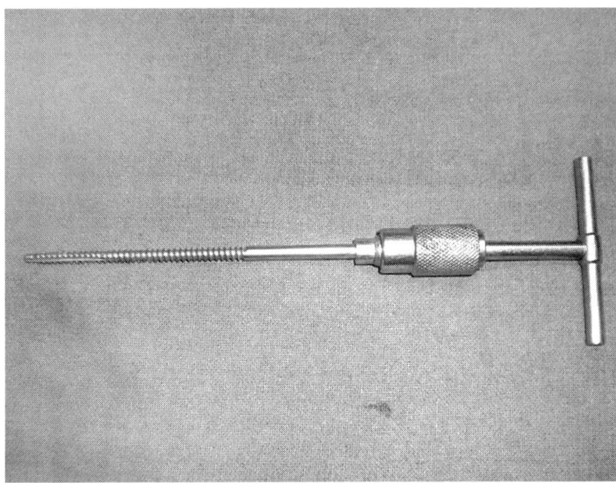

Bone tap key

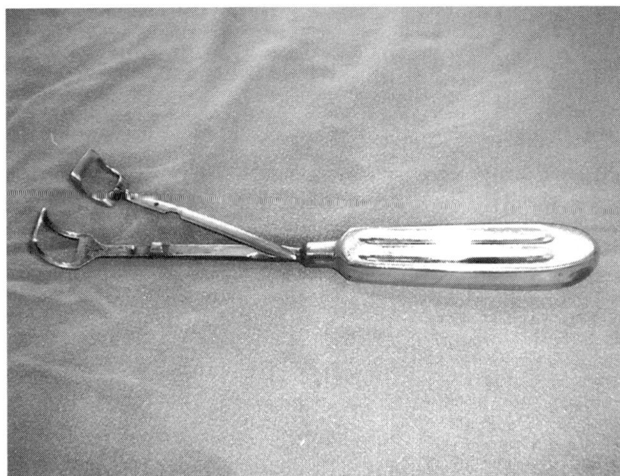

Adenoid curette

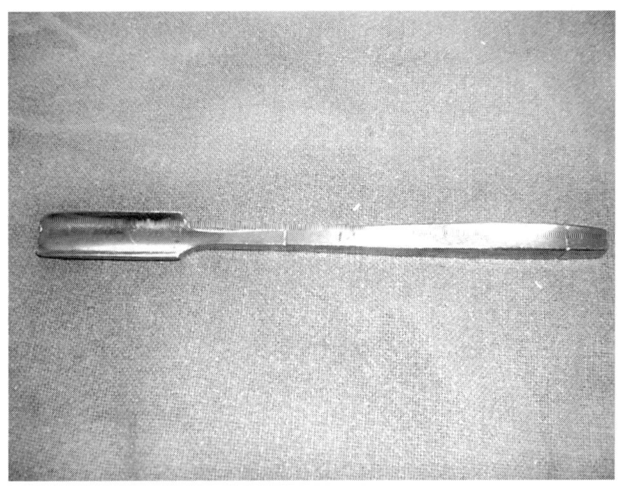

Alexander mastoid gouge

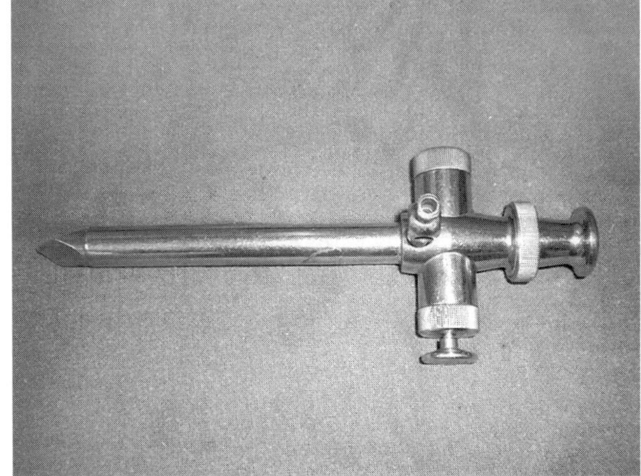

Laparoscope piston valve cannula

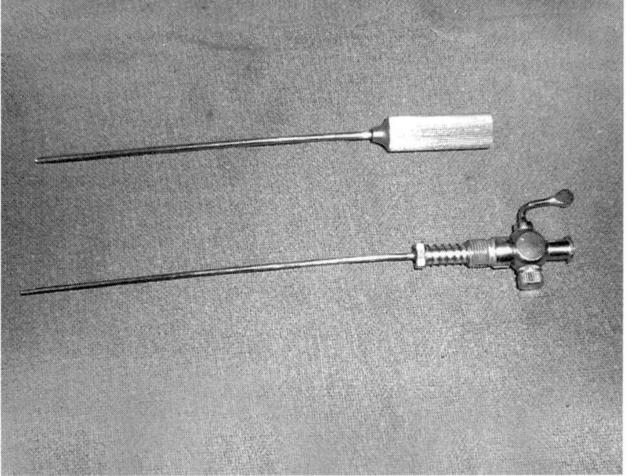

Laparoscope veress needle guard with needle

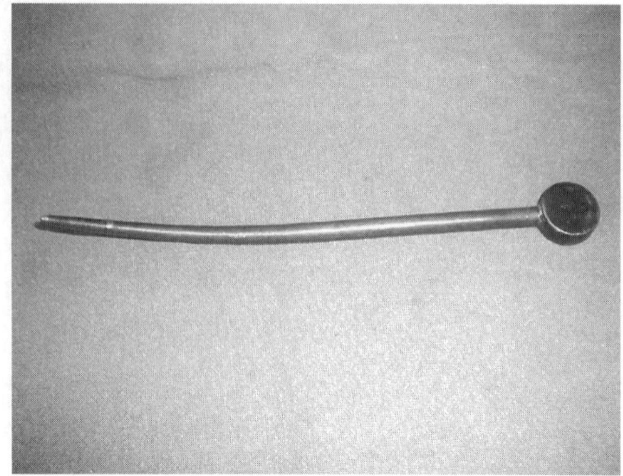

Trocar tunneling instrument

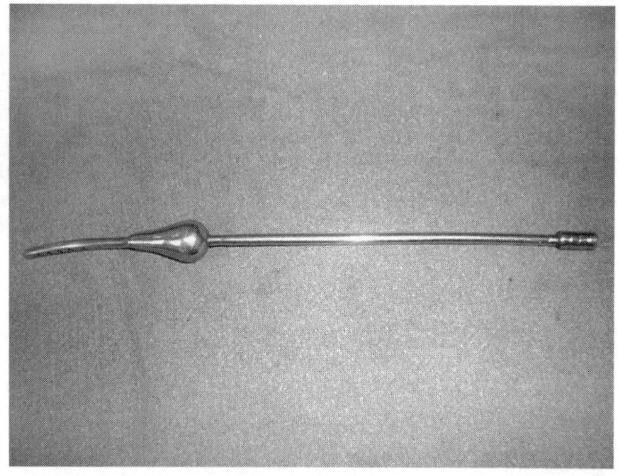

Rubin's cannula

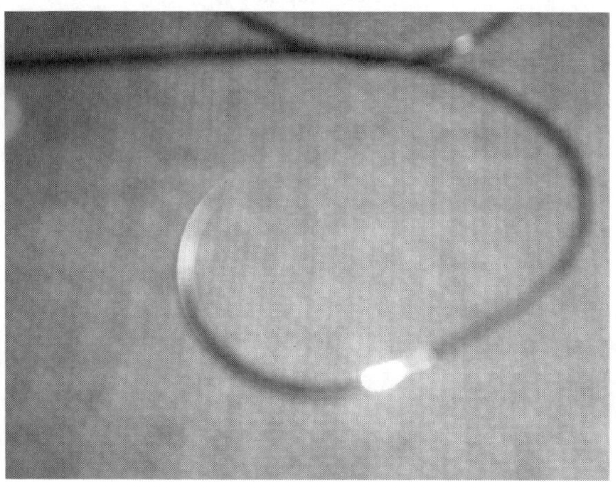

Half-circled round body needle

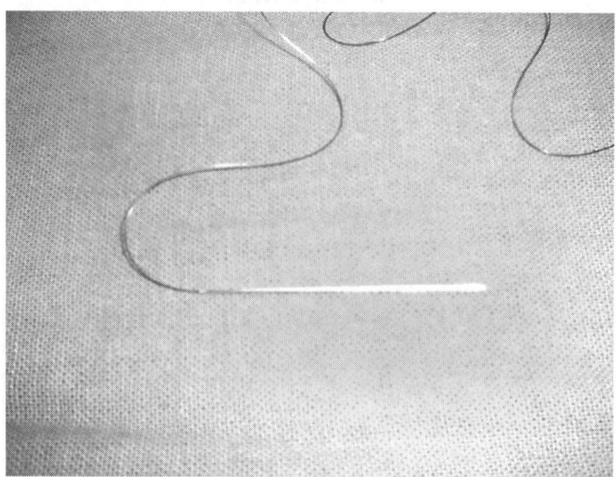

Straight surgical needle

GRASPING INSTRUMENTS

Grasping instruments are the holding instruments as their usable parts are used for tissue retraction. These include tissue forceps, towel clips, tenacula, bone holders, rib approximators, artery forceps, etc.

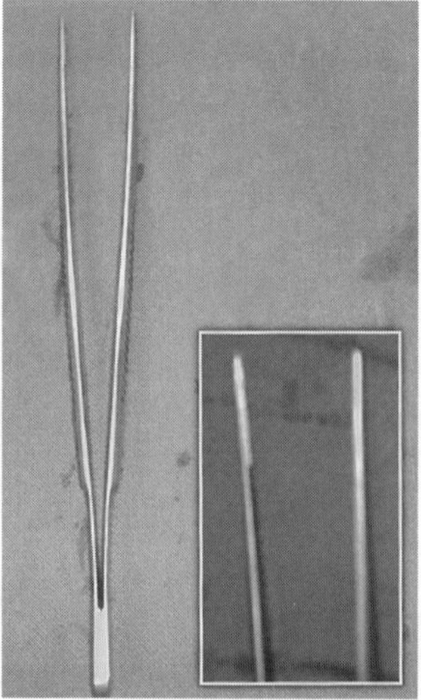

Non-toothed plain forceps

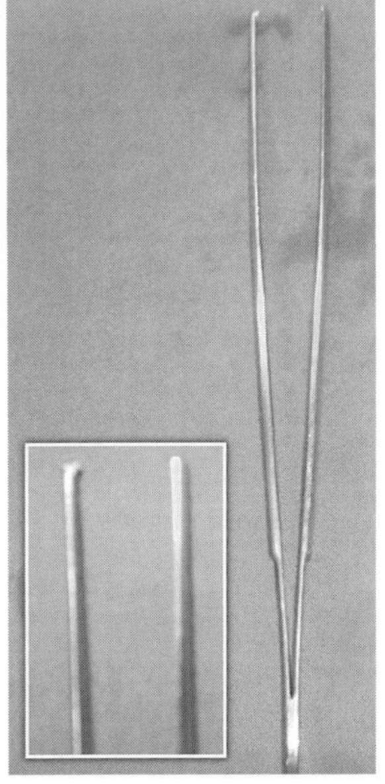

Toothed dissecting forceps

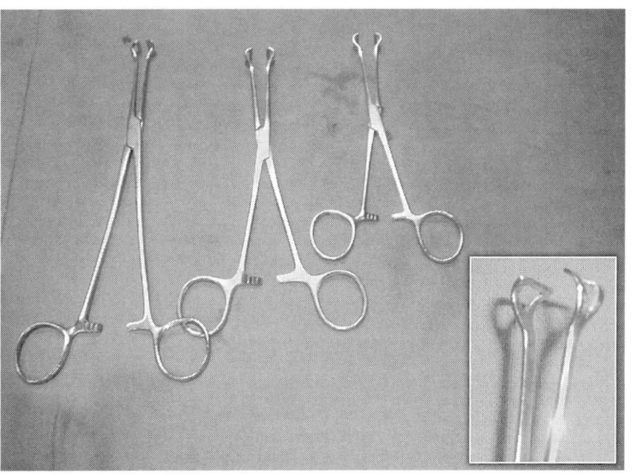

Babcock tissue forceps

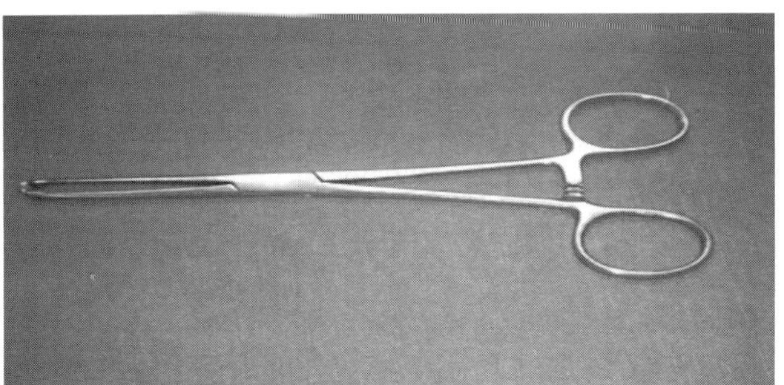

Allis tissue forceps

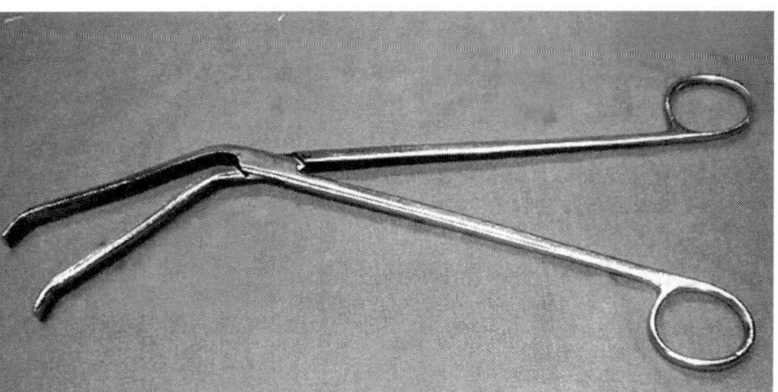

Cheatle forceps

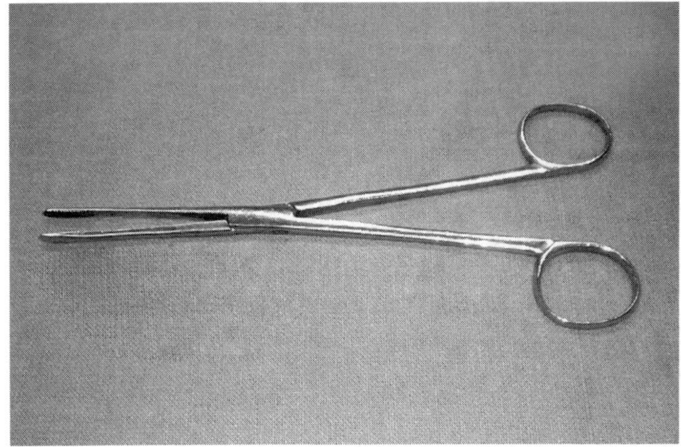

Sinus tissue forceps

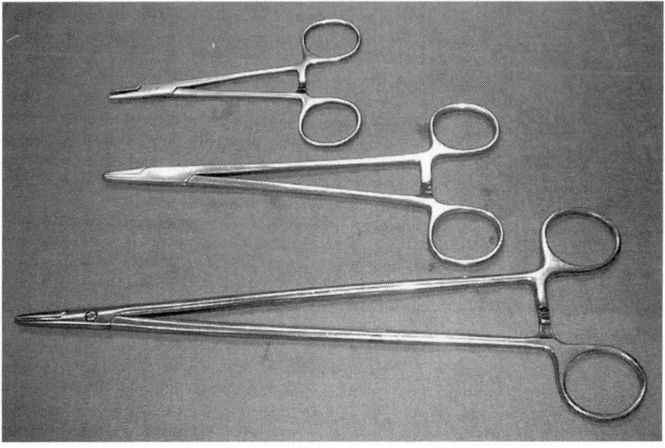

Ayer's needle holder (fine, medium, long)

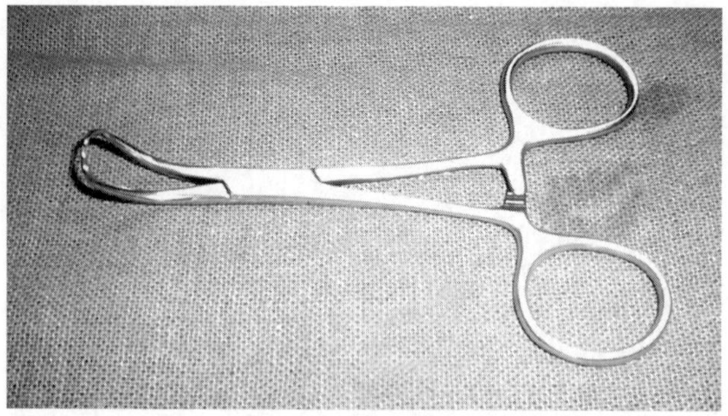
Moynihan's tetra towel clips

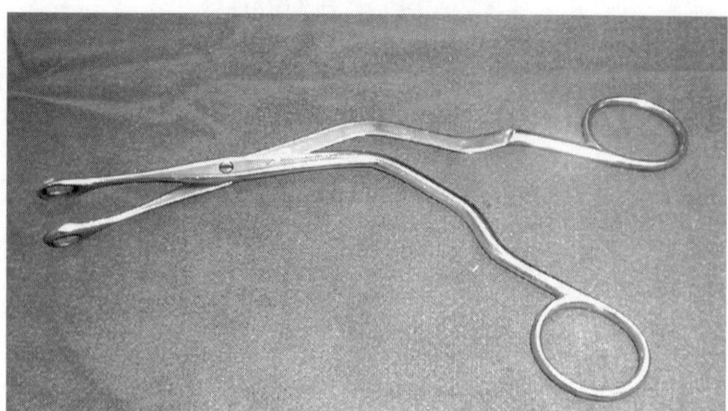
Tonsil forceps

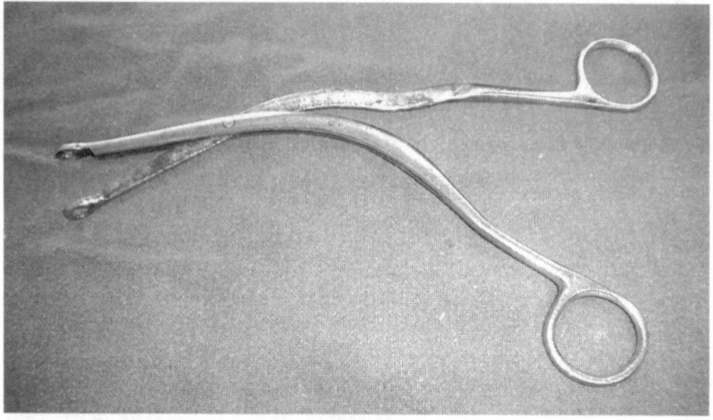
Luc's forceps

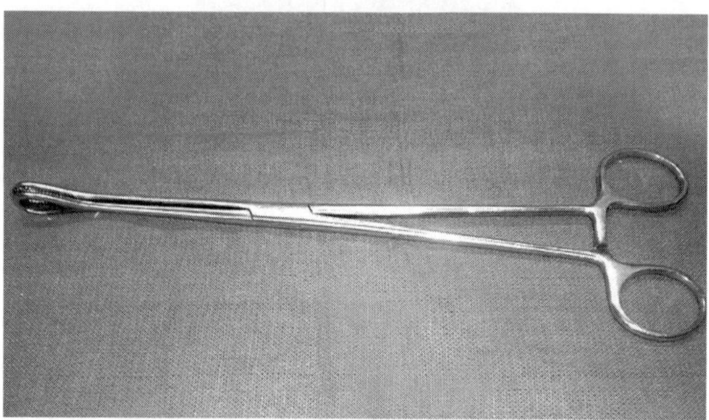
Sponge holder

CLAMPING INSTRUMENTS

Clamping instruments are the ones whose usable parts are generally being used as a method of hemostasis. These instruments are used as graspers or retractors. These include all hemostatic forceps and clamps designed for particular organ like gallbladder forceps, intestinal clamps, blood vessel clamps, and kidney pedicle clamps, etc.

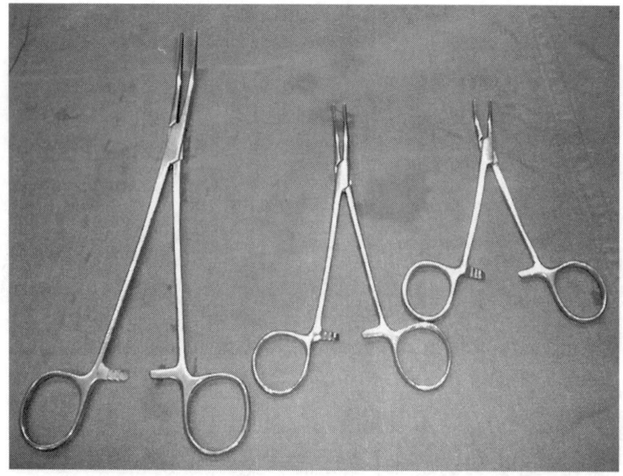
Artery clamp (long, medium, small/mosquito)

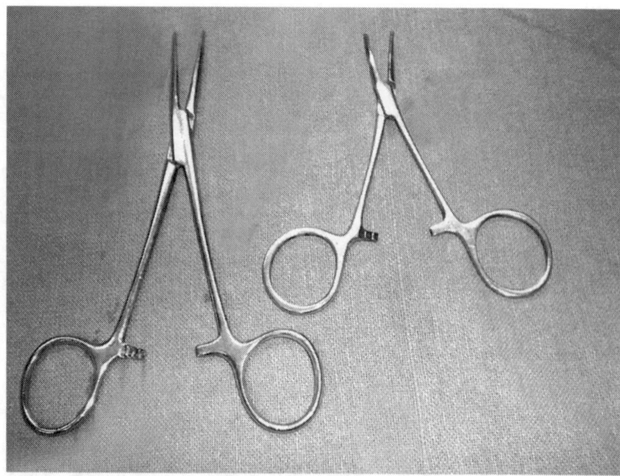
Artery clamp (fine mosquito, baby mixture)

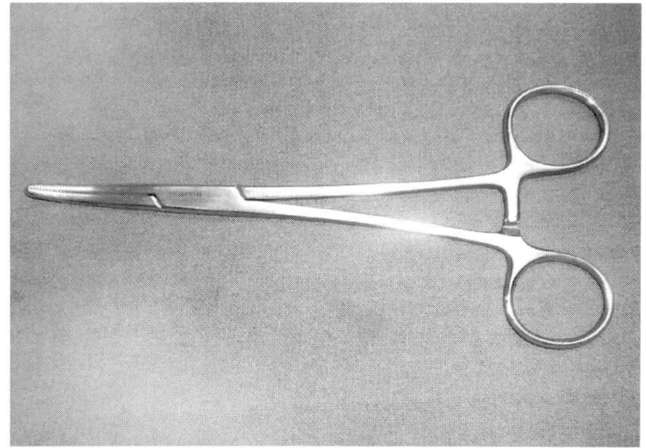

Robert's artery clamp

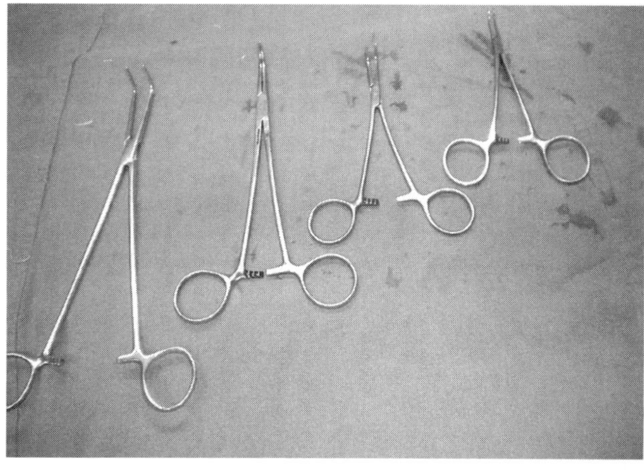

Right angle artery clamp
(long, medium, small, baby mixture)

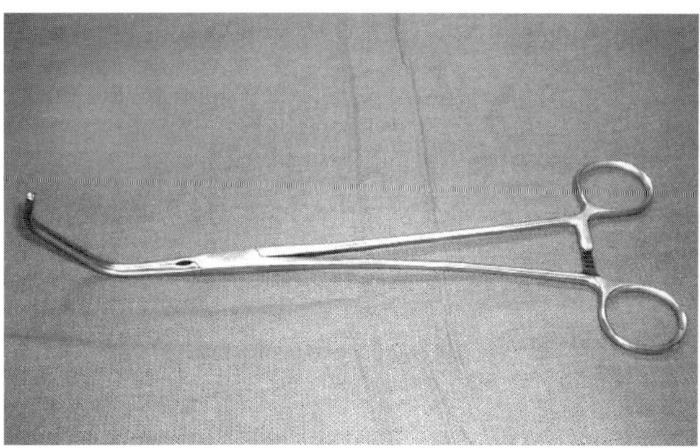

Beck aorta vascular clamp

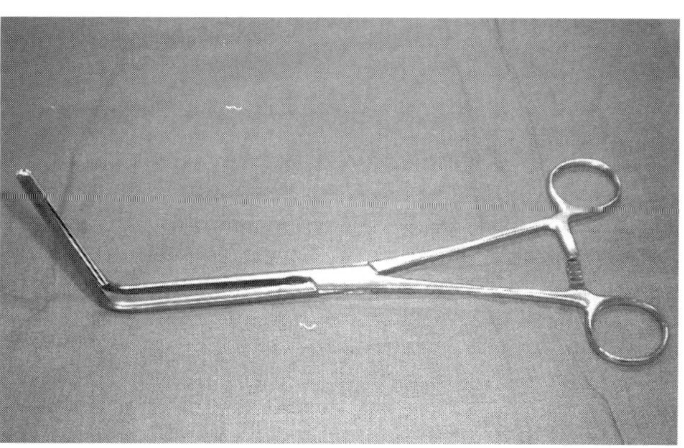

Rectal clamp

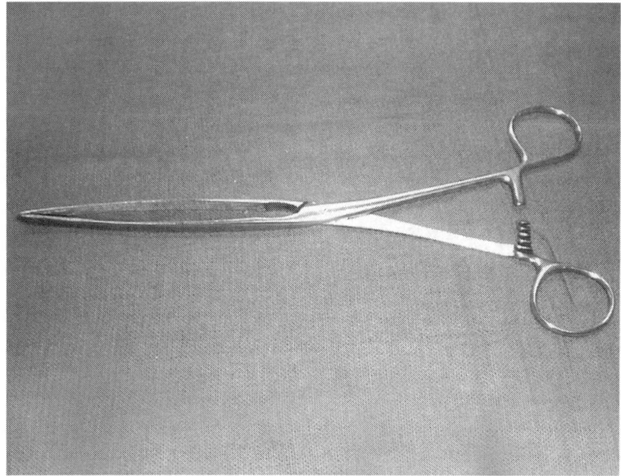

Intestinal clamp—straight

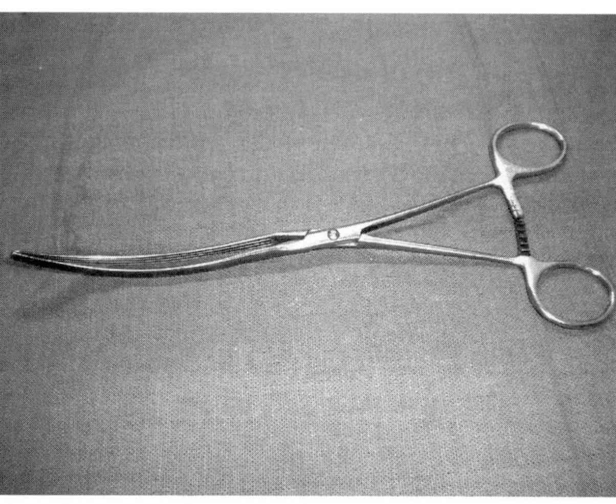

Intestinal clamp—curved

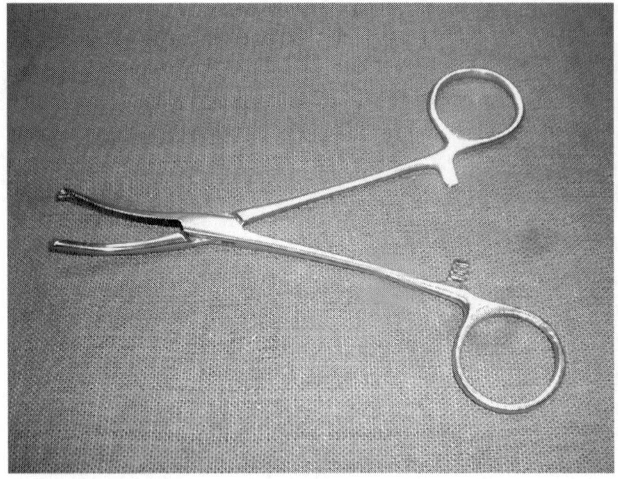
Kocher's clamp

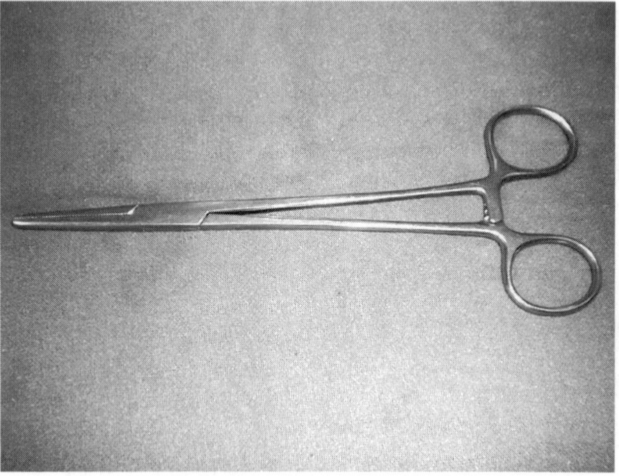
Straight tip long handle clamp

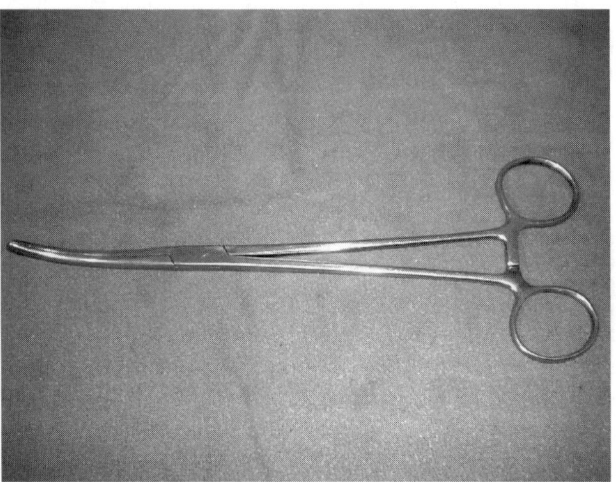
Curved tip long handle clamp

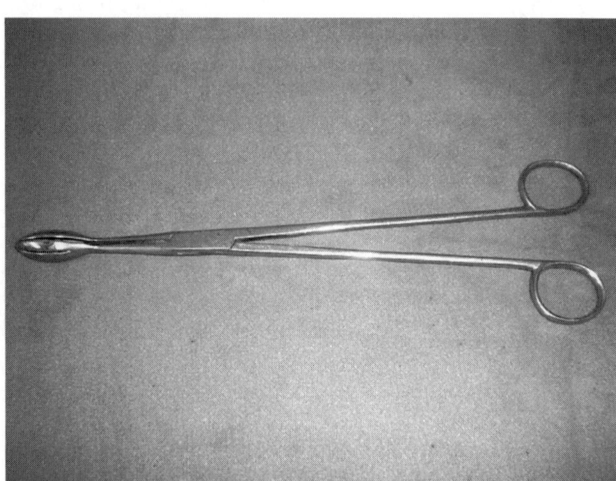
Ovum forceps

EXPOSING INSTRUMENTS

Exposing instruments are used to hold the tissue away from operative site. Few examples are retractors (both self-retaining and manual), specula and endoscopes.

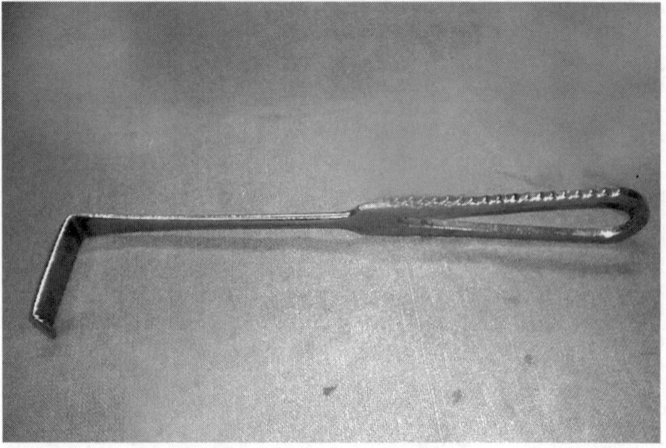
Langenbeck manual retractor

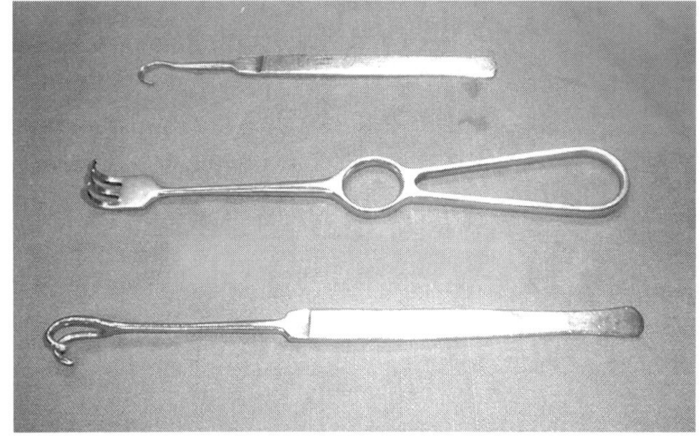

Hook manual retractor (single, multiple hook)

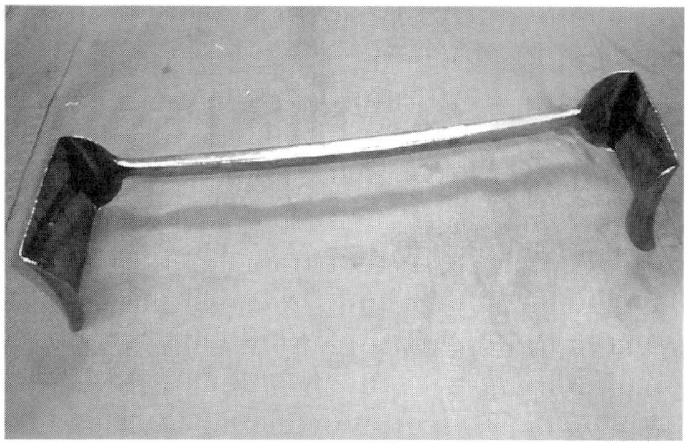

Moris manual retractor

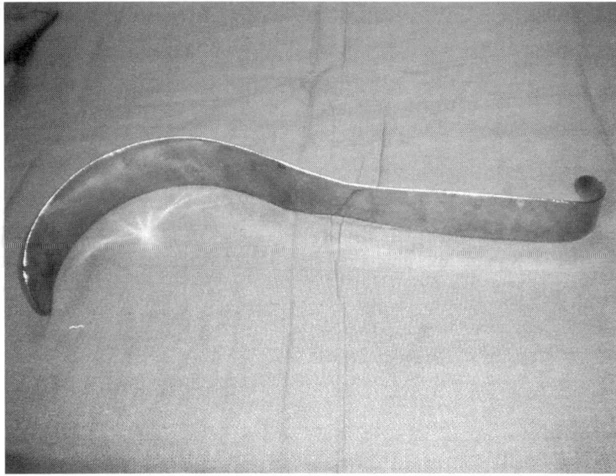

Deaver manual retractor

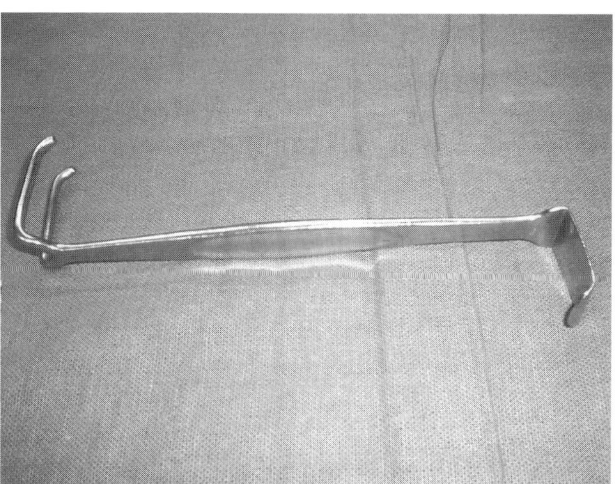

Czerney's manual retractor

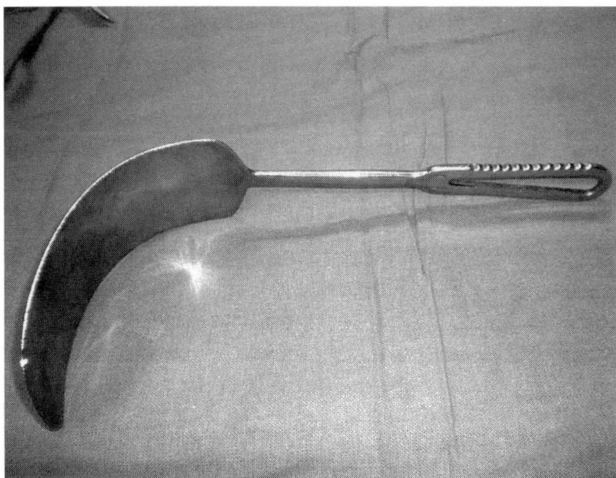

Kelley's manual retractor

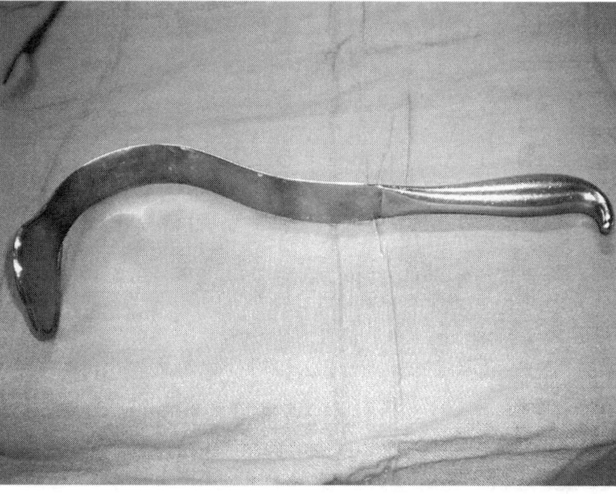

Harrington manual retractor

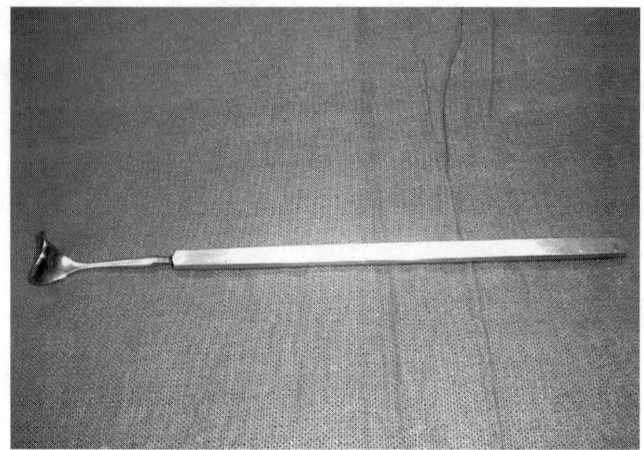
Gil-Vernet manual retractor

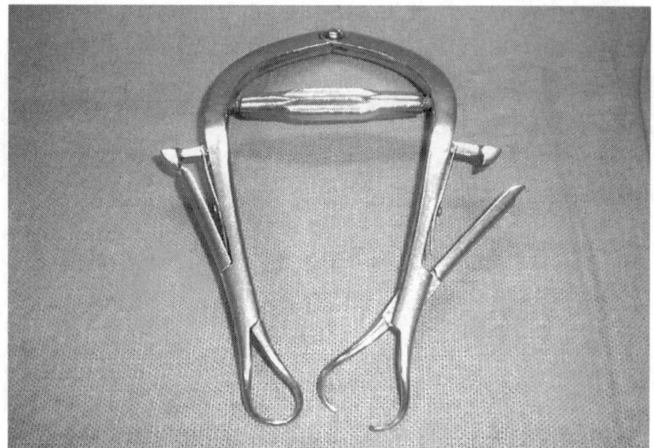
Joule's self-retaining retractor

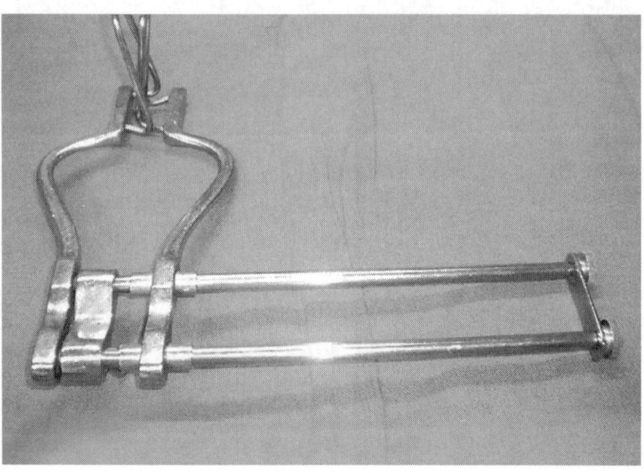
Balfour's self-retaining retractor

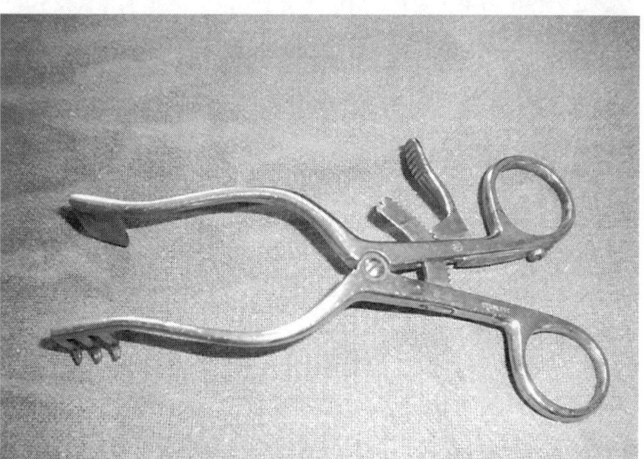
Mastoid self-retaining retractor

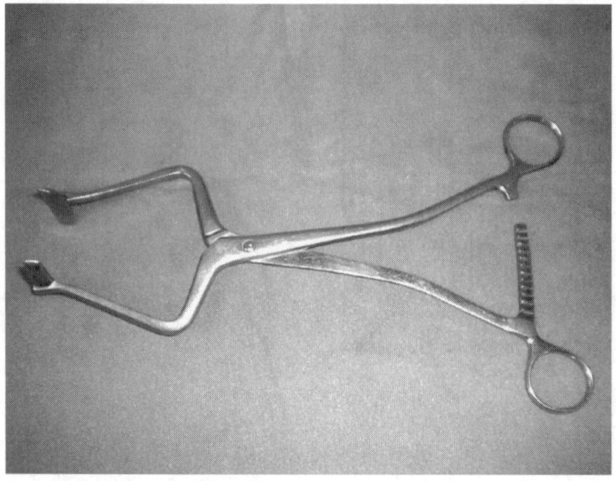
Uterine self-retaining retractor

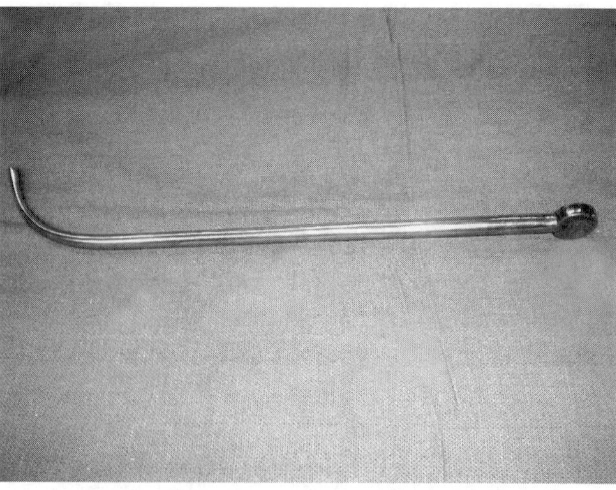
Kollman's, urethral dilator

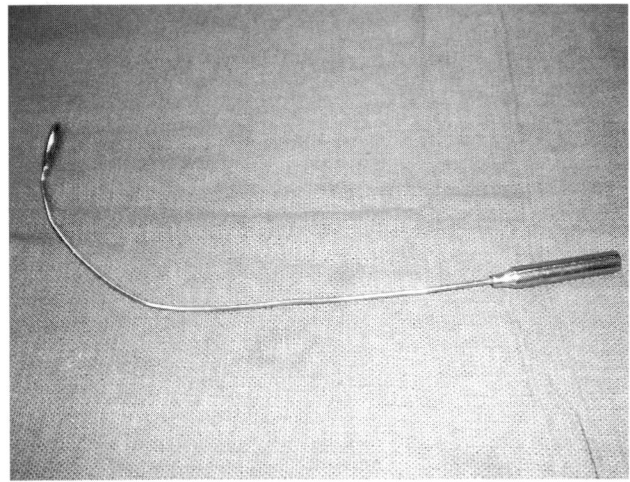
CB duct dilator

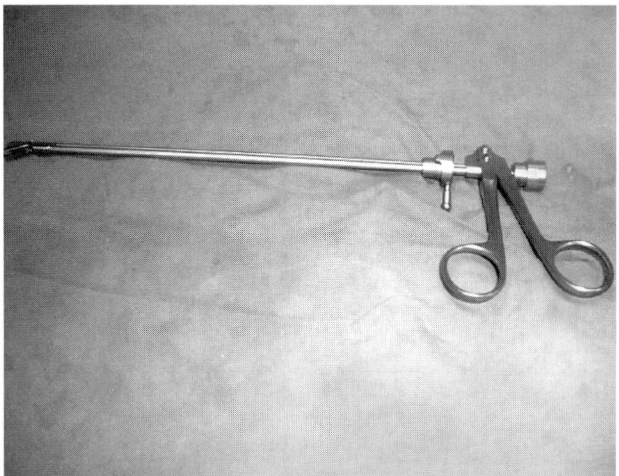
Punch forceps

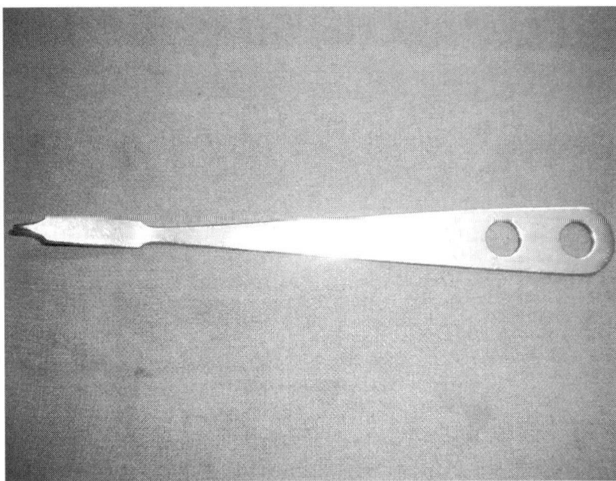
Hoffman

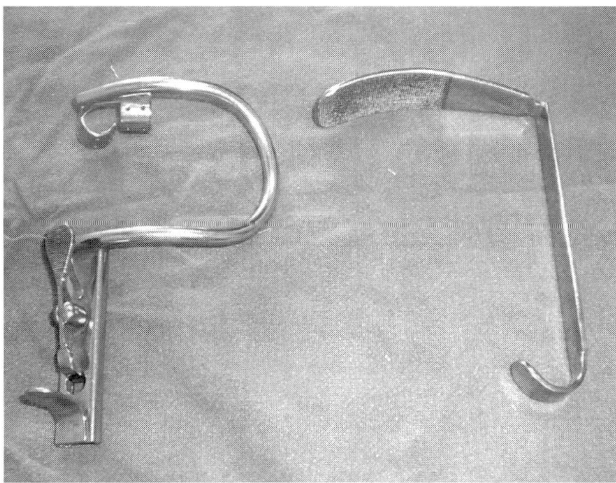
Bowle's Davis mouth gag blade

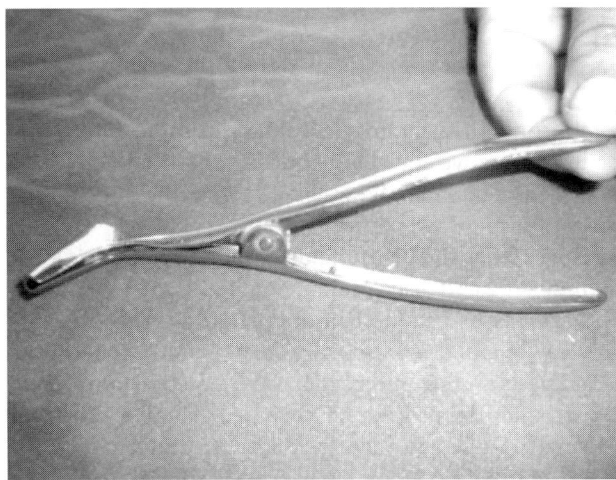
Nasal speculum

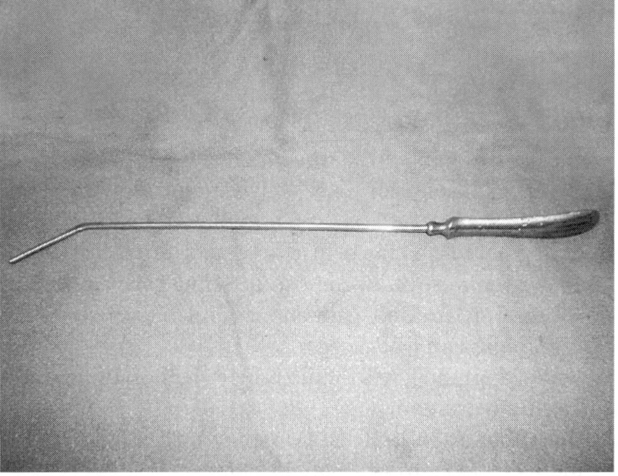
Uterine sound

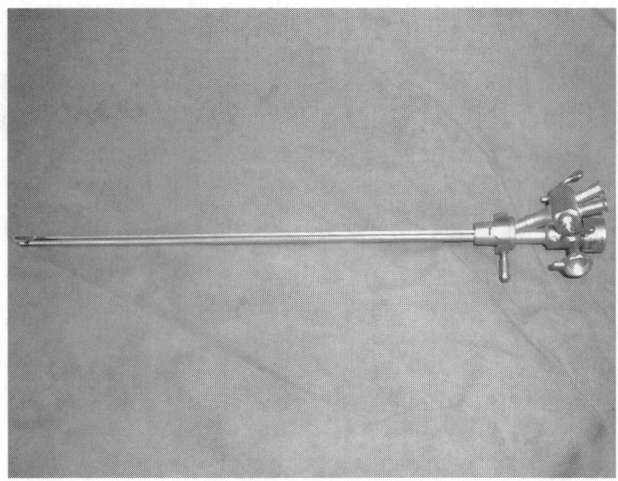

Cystoscope—deflecting channel

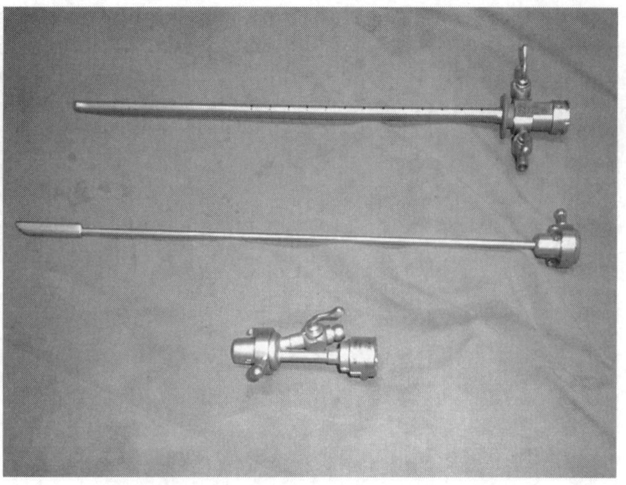

Cystoscope sheath with bridge
(set of 3—sheath, obturator, telescope bridge)

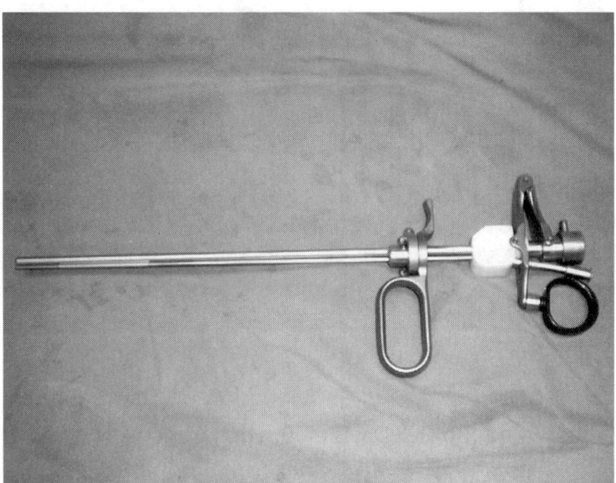

Rectoscope working element

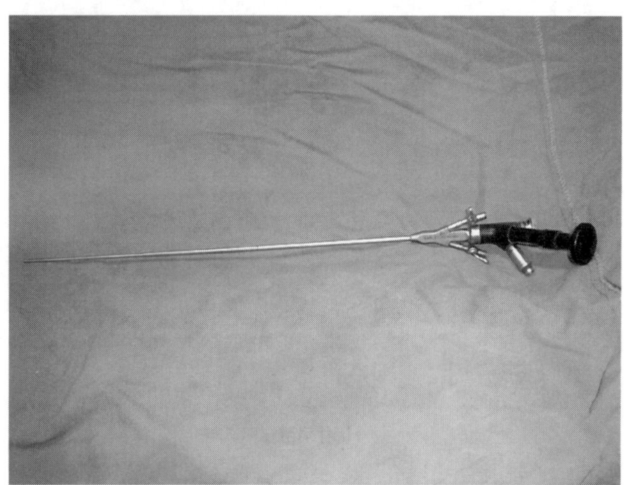

Urethroscope sheath

Care of Instruments

Surgical instruments constitute a high monetary investment and a critical factor for an effective surgical intervention. Therefore, they should be used and maintained very carefully. Regular inspection of instruments is important before and after their usage. Each hospital should have clear cut policy on their care and maintenance and this policy should be understood and followed.

Following guidelines should be used while handling and caring for instruments:

- Instruments shall be used as intended, a damaged instrument can jeopardize a patient's life.
- Rinse the instruments in coldwater immediately after use to remove any blood, mucus.
- Instruments must be washed thoroughly; they do not require any preservatives.
- Never leave the instruments in saline solution, it leads to rusting and discoloration.
- Before storing, instruments should be thoroughly cleaned and dried.
- All parts of instruments must be counted before, during and after the procedure, as some have nuts, screws or small parts which might get dislodged and remain in the client's body.

Nursing Case Study/ Presentation

9

OBJECTIVES

After completion of this chapter, students will be able to:

- Build a scientific knowledge base in using nursing case study/case presentation as a method of patient care.
- Comprehend the significance of nursing case study/case presentation method in patient care.
- Develop beginning skills in conducting an in-depth case study.

NURSING CASE STUDY

Nursing case study method originated many centuries ago when it was adopted by Hippocrates to teach medicine. Even in nursing, case study method has been used more extensively than any other method.

Nursing case study is defined as a thorough description of the life history of a selected patient. It gives an in-depth knowledge of selected case. In nursing case study, student nurse gathers a baseline data of her patient, prepares her own plan of action, implements it, evaluates it under the guidance of her clinical supervisor. This method provides an excellent learning experience for the student as it correlates the patient personality, his needs and nursing care.

The *first* part of the study is concerned with the basic information and facts about the patient, his diagnosis, socioeconomic and personal history and how this data is applied in determining nursing care of this patient.

The *second* part of the study is concerned with comprehensive nursing care of patient. Firstly the student nurse identifies her responsibilities, patient needs and related activities and secondly these activities are documented into a nursing care plan.

Throughout the nursing case study not only the patient's needs are constantly emphasized, but this is also an excellent means for the student nurse to practice her nursing skills.

CASE PRESENTATION

Case/patient presentation requires the presence of selected patient with entire focus on discussion of his diseased condition and related care. Case presentation method provides an opportunity to the students nurses to view the actual patient problems and strengthen their ability to see the relationship between patient's health status, his problems, and how the solution to these problems could be arrived at.

An effective case presentation requires:

a. Selection of a case
b. Patient consent
c. Selecting the setting – at bedside or clinical classroom
d. Advance preparation of the student nurse

In case presentation although patient's diseased condition is briefly discussed, but the major emphasis is on nursing care.

Criteria for Case Study/Case Presentation

- Minimum five days of continuous nursing care.
- Daily evaluation of objectives.

Gadgets Used in ICU

10

OBJECTIVES

After completion of this chapter, students will be able to:

- Identify the gadgets in ICU.
- Describe how these gadgets affect patient condition
- Describe nursing care of their patients.
- Evaluate the effectiveness of these gadgets.
- Identify emergency interventions for critically ill patients.

INTRODUCTION

An Intensive Care Unit (ICU), also known as an Intensive Therapy Unit or Intensive Treatment Unit (ITU) or Critical Care Unit (CCU), is a special department of a hospital or health care facility that provides intensive care medicine.

Intensive care units cater to patients with the most severe and life-threatening illnesses and injuries which require constant, close invasive monitoring and support from specialist equipment and medication in order to ensure normal bodily functions. They are staffed by highly trained doctors and critical care nurses who specialize in caring for seriously ill patients. Common conditions that are treated within ICUs include trauma, multiple organ failure and sepsis.

Patients may be transferred directly to an intensive care unit from an emergency department if required, or from a ward if they rapidly deteriorate, or immediately after surgery if the surgery is very invasive and the patient is at high-risk of complications (Fig. 10.1).

How is ICU different from other hospital units?

Care in the ICU differs from other hospital units as:

- Seriously ill patients require close observation and monitoring. Specially trained nurses care for one or two patients at a time, each shift. ICU doctors are specially trained critical care doctors.
- Patients may have special equipment in their room, depending on their unique situation and condition. The equipment in the ICU may seem overwhelming. Patients are connected to machines to monitor their heart, blood pressure, and respiratory rate. Ventilators (breathing machines) assist some patients with breathing until they are able to breathe on their own.

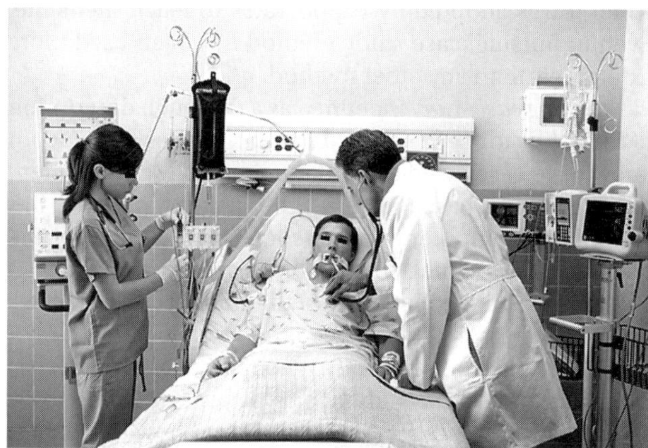

Fig. 10.1: Patient in ICU

HEALTH TEAM MEMBERS OF ICU

- Intensive care nurse
- Intensive care doctors
- **Other intensive care team members:** Ward clerk provide administrative assistance for the ICU team orderly/wards person/patient care assistant—these staff assist nurses with patient care including turns and mobility as well as transfers to other areas of the hospital (Fig. 10.2A and B).
- **Allied health professionals:** The ICU team cannot care for the ICU patient without the help of other health care professionals. Within the ICU there are other members like:
- **Physiotherapists:** They are responsible for providing physical therapy for patients such as mobility assistance and chest physiotherapy.

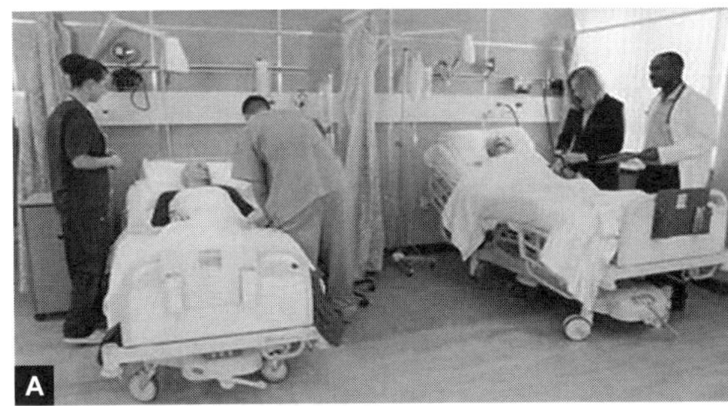

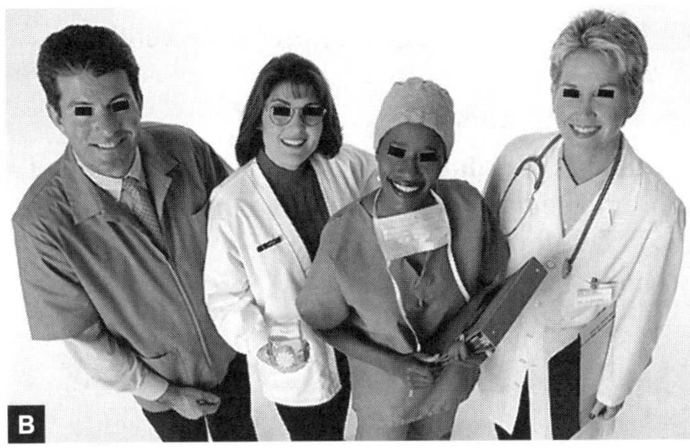

Figs. 10.2A and B: Team members of ICU

- **Pharmacists:** They attend ward rounds and assist doctors and nurses with advice regarding medications as well as ensuring a supply of medication for patients.
- **Social workers:** They are available at most large hospitals. They provide invaluable support for families of critically ill including counseling and assistance with financial matters.
- **Occupational therapists:** They evaluate the ability of the patient to carry out everyday activities of daily leaving and develop treatment plans to improve the patient's abilities.
- **Speech therapists:** They evaluate the speech and swallowing of patients.
- **Dietitians:** They provide advice on the best nutrition for patients.
- **Radiography technicians**.

RESPONSIBILITIES OF AN ICU NURSE

Intensive care unit nurses or critical care nurses are registered nurses who specialize in providing care in intensive care units of hospitals. An ICU nurse assess, plan, implement and evaluate health care services for patients suffering with a broad range of health conditions. Nurses in general intensive care units commonly provide care to patients suffering from cardiac disease and brain injuries. Accident victims and patients recuperating from complex surgeries frequently need nursing care from critical care specialists as well. ICU nurses work closely with physicians and other members of the health care team. They need to be skilled in assessment of patients and capable of using high tech equipment. It must possess physical, mental, and emotional stamina to work with seriously ill patients and their loved ones.

- They calculate medication doses and titrate potent medications.
- They insert and care for specialized venous and arterial infusions.
- They must be adept at mathematics and the use ventilators and other high tech equipment.
- They care for dying patients and provide education and support to family members faced with critical decisions such as discontinuing life support and deciding how to care for people with brain injuries.

GADGETS USED IN ICU

Intensive care unit equipment includes patient monitoring, respiratory and cardiac support, pain management, emergency resuscitation devices, and other life support equipment designed to care for patients who are seriously injured, have a critical or life-threatening illness, or have undergone a major surgical procedure, thereby requiring 24-hour care and monitoring.

Purpose

An ICU may be designed and equipped to provide care to patients with a range of conditions or it may be designed and equipped to provide specialized care to patients with specific conditions. For example, a neuromedical ICU cares for patients with acute conditions involving the nervous system or patients who have just had neurosurgical procedures and require equipment for monitoring and assessing the brain and spinal cord. A neonatal ICU is designed and equipped to care for infants who are ill born prematurely or have a condition requiring constant monitoring. A trauma/burn ICU provides specialized injury and wound care for patients involved in auto accidents and patients who have gunshot injuries or burns.

Intensive care unit equipment includes patient monitoring, life support and emergency resuscitation devices and diagnostic devices. There are ventilator, defibrillators, cardiac monitor; various tubes like endotracheal tube, nasogastric tube, etc. crash cart, catheters and infusion pump. We will discuss about all equipment in detail.

VENTILATORS

A medical ventilator (or simply ventilator in context) is a machine designed to mechanically move breathable air into and out of the lungs, to provide the mechanism of breathing for a patient who is physically unable to breathe, or breathing insufficiently. (Fig. 10.3) Mechanical ventilation is a method to mechanically assist or replace spontaneous breathing. Mechanical ventilation is termed 'invasive' if it involves any instrument penetrating through the mouth (such as an endotracheal tube) or the skin (such as a tracheostomy tube).

Mechanical ventilation is indicated when the patient's spontaneous ventilation is inadequate to maintain life (Fig. 10.4). It is also indicated as prophylaxis for imminent collapse of other physiologic functions, or ineffective gas exchange in the lungs. Because mechanical ventilation serves only to provide assistance for breathing and does not cure a disease, the patient's underlying condition should be correctable and should resolve over time.

Indications

- Acute lung injury [including Acute Respiratory Distress Syndrome (ARDS), trauma].
- Apnea with respiratory arrest including cases from intoxication.
- Acute severe asthma, requiring intubation.
- Chronic Obstructive Pulmonary Disease (COPD).

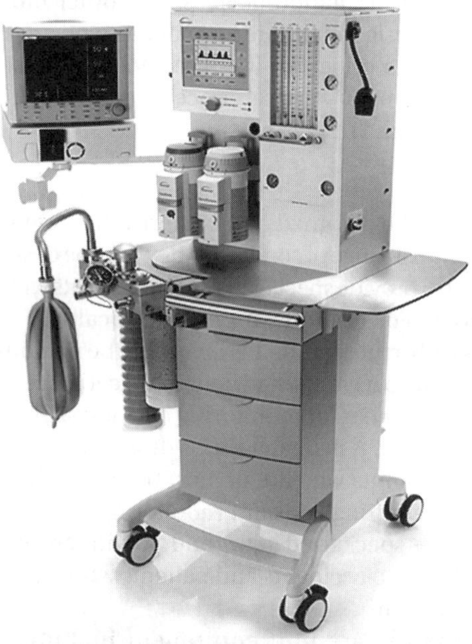

Fig. 10.3: Medical ventilation

- Acute respiratory acidosis with partial pressure of carbon dioxide (PCO_2) > 50 mm Hg and pH < 7.25.
- Increased work of breathing as evidenced by significant tachypnea, retractions, and other physical signs of respiratory distress.
- Hypoxemia with arterial partial pressure of oxygen (PO_2) < 55 mm Hg with supplemental fraction of inspired oxygen (FiO_2) = 1.0.
- Hypotension including sepsis, shock, congestive heart failure.
- Neurological diseases such as muscular dystrophy and amyotrophic lateral sclerosis.

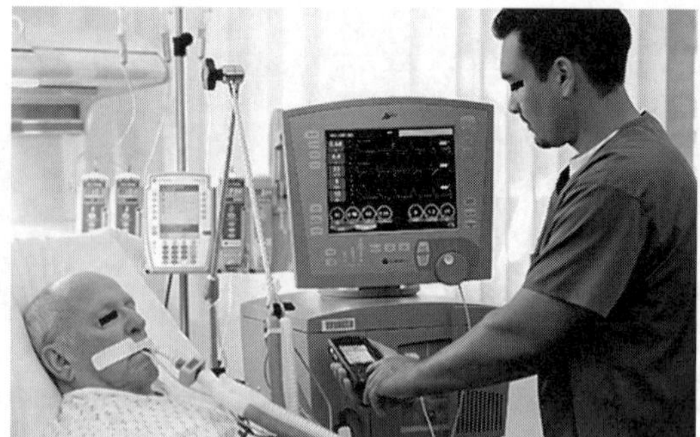

Fig. 10.4: High frequency oscillation ventilator

Types of Ventilators

- **Transport ventilators:** These ventilators are small and more rugged and can be powered pneumatically or via AC or DC power sources (Fig. 10.5).

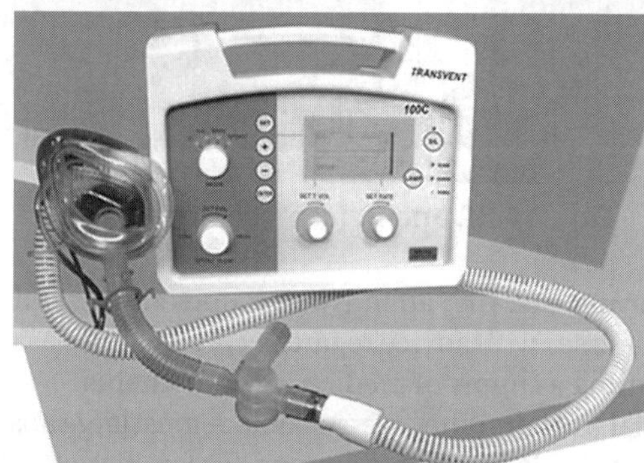

Fig. 10.5: Transport ventilator

- **Intensive-care ventilators:** These ventilators are larger and usually run on AC power (though virtually all contain a battery to facilitate intrafacility transport and as a backup in the event of a power failure). This style of ventilator often provides greater control of a wide variety of ventilation parameters (such as inspiratory rise time). Many ICU ventilators also incorporate graphics to provide visual feedback of each breath.
- **Neonatal ventilators:** Designed with the preterm neonate in mind, these are a specialized subset of ICU ventilators that are designed to deliver the smaller, more precise volumes and pressures required to ventilate these patients.
- **Positive airway pressure (PAP) ventilators:** These ventilators are specifically designed for non-invasive ventilation. This includes ventilators for use at home for the treatment of chronic conditions such as sleep apnea or COPD.

We usually use positive airway pressure ventilators in our hospitals. Three basic types of positive pressure ventilators are as follows:

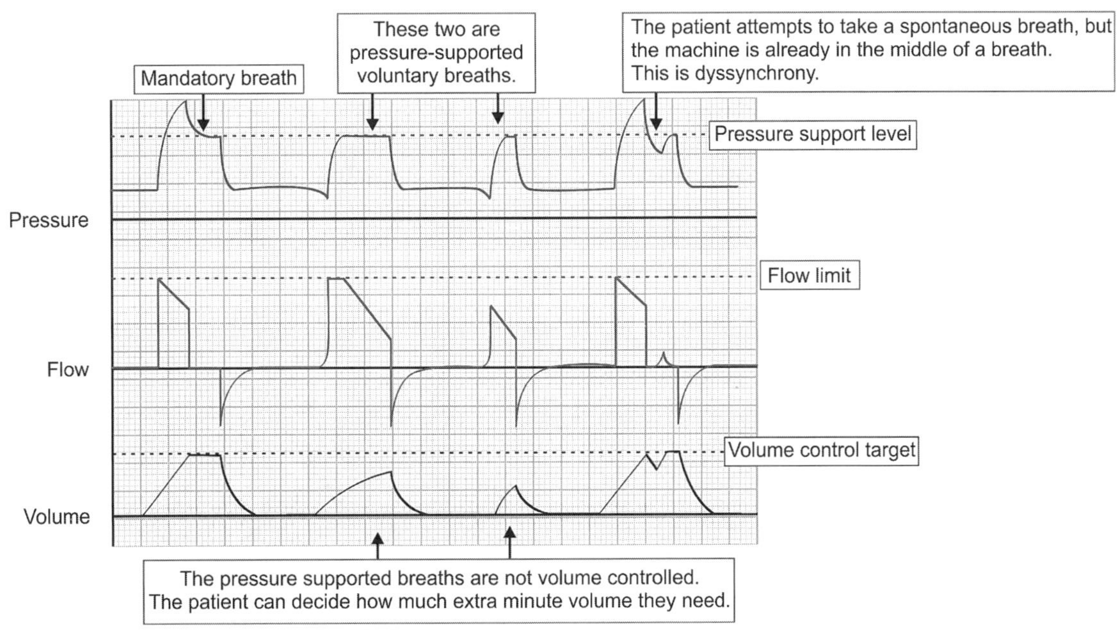

Fig. 10.6: Respiratory patterns-pressure supported

1. **Pressure-cycled ventilation:** Deliver a volume of gas to the airway using position pressure during inspiration. This positive pressure is delivered until reselected pressure has been reached. When the preset pressure is reached, the machine cycle into exhalation. Pressure cycled is used only in a small portion of client who require CMV.
2. **Volume-cycled ventilation (volume-controlled or volume-limited):** Deliver a preset that has been reselected is delivered this volume. A pressure limit can be set to prevent the occurrence of dangerously high airway pressure.
3. **Time-cycled ventilation:** Terminate when preset inspiratory time has elapsed. In most of these devices, a pressure limit is also incorporated.

Modes of Ventilation

Modes of ventilation refer to the way the client receives breaths from ventilators. There are several conventional methods of continuous mechanical ventilators.

Volume Mode (Fig. 10.7)

- **Control mode:** It is independent of client's effort or pattern of breathing. The machine is set for automatic operation and for producing a set number of cycles per minute at a predetermined flow rate. This mode is used only when the client cannot make any respiratory effort or is chemically paralyzed with neuromuscular blocking agents such as neuron or pancuronium bromide.
- **Assist control mode:** The inspiratory phase of the respirator's cycle is triggered by the patient's spontaneous inspiration. It may either compliment the patient's ventilator volume or augment his respiration with a preset rate of ventilation. These are mostly equipped with safety function so that if patient's respiratory function fails to trigger the ventilator by a preset interval of time, the control ventilation automatically takes over.

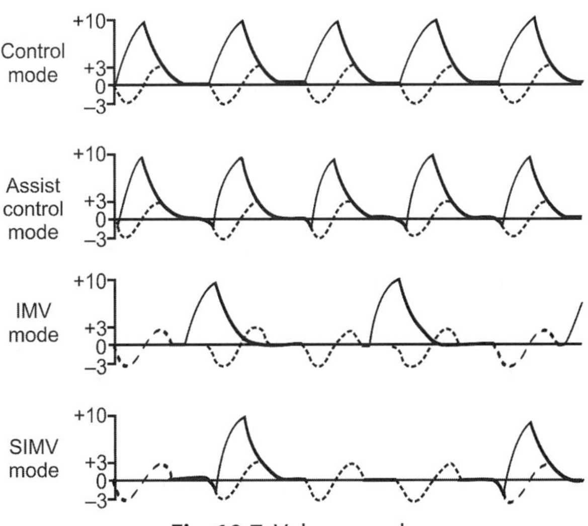

Fig. 10.7: Volume mode

- **Synchronized intermittent-mandatory ventilation (SIMV):** Guarantees a certain number of breaths, but unlike ACV, patient breaths are partially their own, reducing the risk of hyperinflation or alkalosis. Mandatory breaths are synchronized to coincide with spontaneous respirations. Disadvantages of SIMV are increased work of breathing and a tendency to reduce cardiac output which may prolong ventilator dependency. The addition of pressure support on top of spontaneous breaths can reduce some of the work of breathing. SIMV has been shown to decrease cardiac output in patients with left-ventricular dysfunction.

Pressure Mode

- Less risk of barotrauma as compared to ACV and SIMV does not allow for patient-initiated breaths. The inspiratory flow pattern decreases exponentially, reducing peak pressures and improving gas exchange. The major disadvantage is that there are no guarantees for volume, especially when lung mechanics are changing. Thus, PCV has traditionally been preferred for patients with neuromuscular disease but otherwise normal lungs.
- **Pressure support ventilation (PSV):** Allows the patient to determine inflation volume and respiratory frequency (but not pressure, as this is pressure-controlled), thus can only be used to augment spontaneous breathing. Pressure support can be used to overcome the resistance of ventilator tubing in another cycle (5–10 cm, H_2O are generally used, especially during weaning), or to augment spontaneous breathing. It can be delivered through specialized face masks.
- **Pressure controlled inverse ratio ventilation (PCIRV):** Pressure controlled ventilatory mode in which the majority of time is spent at the higher (inspiratory) pressure. Early trials were promising, however, the risks of auto PEEP and hemodynamic deterioration due to the decreased expiratory time and increased mean airway pressure generally outweighs the small potential for improved oxygenation.
- **Airway pressure release ventilation (APRV):** Airway pressure release ventilation is similar to PCIRV—instead of being a variation of PCV in which the I:E ratio is reversed; APRV is a variation of CPAP that releases pressure temporarily on exhalation. This unique mode of ventilation results in higher average airway pressures. Patients are able to spontaneously ventilate at both low and high pressures, although typically most or all ventilation occurs at the high pressure.

Weaning

Weaning refers to the process in which intensive care staff tries to get a patient to breathe without the help of the mechanical ventilator (Fig. 10.8). When patients have recovered enough, they often can breathe by themselves or with only a little help from the ventilator. This ability is checked during a short testing period called a 'weaning trial.' If the patient remains comfortable during a trial, a small amount of blood may be drawn at the end of the trial to check the level of oxygen and carbon dioxide. If these levels look good, the breathing tube can usually be removed from the lungs. If a patient becomes very short of breath or anxious during the weaning trial or if the levels of oxygen or carbon dioxide are not at an acceptable level, we say that the patient 'failed' the trial. Further attempts at weaning may be made later that day or on another day.

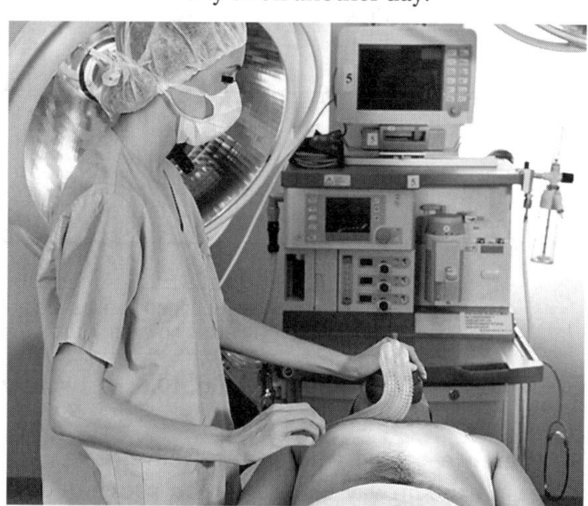

Fig. 10.8: Weaning

In some cases, the intensive care staff chooses to reduce in steps the amount of help a patient gets from the ventilator. This reduction can occur rapidly (over minutes or hours) in patients who are doing well, or it can occur gradually (over days) in patients who are still moderately ill. At each step, the comfort of the patient is assessed.

Nursing Responsibilities

Review Communication

Communication among care providers promotes optimal outcomes. For mechanically ventilated patients, care providers may include primary care physicians, pulmonary specialists, respiratory therapists, and nurses. To make sure you are aware of other team members' communications about the patient, find out the goals of therapy for your patient when obtaining report.

Check Ventilator Settings and Modes

When you enter the patient's room, take vital signs, check oxygen saturation, listen to breath sounds, and note changes from previous findings. Also assess the patient's pain and anxiety levels. Read the patient's order and obtain information about the ventilator. Compare current ventilator settings with the settings prescribed in the order. Familiarize yourself with ventilator alarms and the actions to take when an alarm sounds.

Suction

Patients receiving positive-pressure mechanical ventilation have a tracheostomy, endotracheal, or nasotracheal tube. Most initially have an endotracheal tube if they stay on the ventilator for many days or weeks, a tracheotomy may be done. Suction only as needed—not according to a schedule. Hyperoxygenate the patient before and after suctioning to help prevent oxygen desaturation.

Assess Pain and Sedation Needs

Even though patient cannot verbally express his needs, nurse needs to assess his pain level using a reliable scale. Keep in mind that a patient's acknowledgment of pain means pain is present and must be treated. It is best to treat agitation and anxiety with medication and non-pharmacologic methods such as communication, touch, presence of family members, music, guided imagery, and distraction.

Prevent Infection

Follow all infection control measures to combat infection in ICU.

Prevent Hemodynamic Instability

Monitor the patient's blood pressure every 2 to 4 hours, especially after ventilator settings are changed or adjusted. To maintain hemodynamic stability, you may need to increase intravenous (IV) fluids or administer a drug such as dopamine or norepinephrine, if ordered.

Nutritional Needs

For optimal outcomes, ventilator patients must be well nourished and should begin taking nutrition early. But like any patient who cannot swallow normally, they need an alternative nutrition route. Preferably, they should have feeding tubes with liquid nutrition provided through the gut.

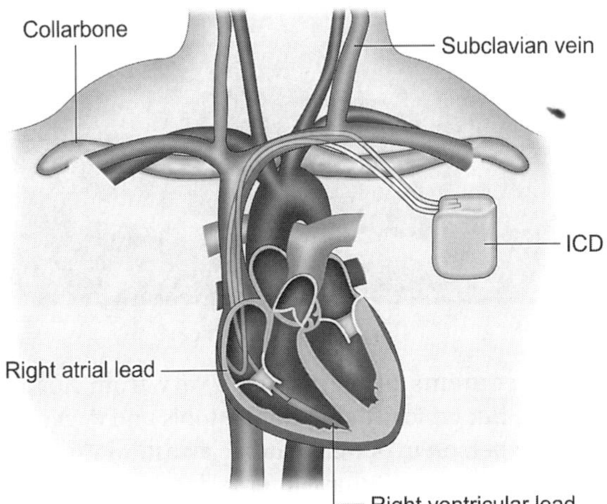

Fig. 10.9: Internal cardiac defibrillator

Patient and Family Education

Seeing a loved one attached to a mechanical ventilator is frightening. To ease distress in the patient and family, teach them why mechanical ventilation is needed and emphasize the positive outcomes it can provide. It is important that the family members take part in patient's care so that they may understand the patient's condition. In this way they will be able to take right decisions regarding the patient's health and also in emergency conditions.

DEFIBRILLATOR

It is a common treatment for life-threatening cardiac dysrhythmias, ventricular fibrillation and pulseless ventricular tachycardia. Defibrillation consists of delivering a therapeutic dose of electrical energy to the heart with a device called a defibrillator. (Fig. 10.10) This depolarizes a critical mass of the heart muscle, terminates the dysrhythmia and allows normal sinus rhythm to be reestablished by the body's natural pacemaker in the sinoatrial node of the heart. Defibrillators can be external, transvenous, or implanted (implantable cardioverter-defibrillator), depending on the type of device used or needed.

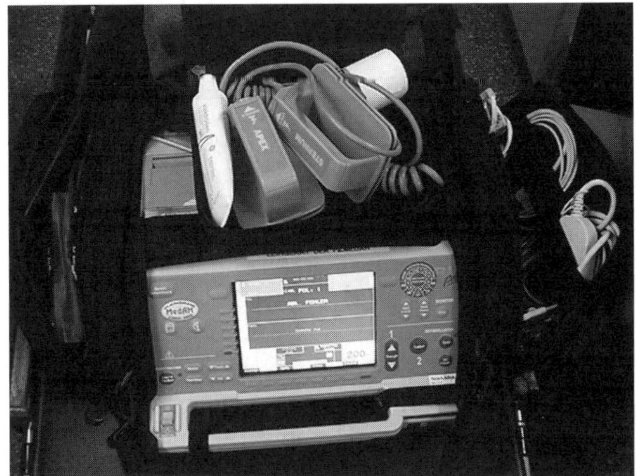

Fig. 10.10: Defibrillator

Types of Defibrillators

- **External defibrillator:** The units are used in conjunction with electrocardiogram readers, which the health care provider uses to diagnose a cardiac condition. The health care provider will then decide what charge (in joules) to use, based on proven guidelines and experience, and will deliver the shock through paddles or pads on the patient's chest. As they require detailed medical knowledge, these units are generally only found in hospitals and on some ambulances.
- **Implanted defibrillator:** It is also known as Automatic Internal Cardiac Defibrillator (AICD). These devices are

implants, similar to pacemakers. They constantly monitor the patient's heart rhythm, and automatically administer shocks for various life-threatening arrhythmias. Many modern devices can distinguish between ventricular fibrillation, ventricular tachycardia, and more benign arrhythmias like supraventricular tachycardia and atrial fibrillation.

- **Wearable defibrillator:** A wearable defibrillator straps on to the outside of the patient to provide continuous monitoring through non-adhesive electrodes. (Fig. 10.11) Like the implantable defibrillator, this device detects an abnormal heart rhythm and can deliver a shock to restore a normal heart rhythm. It provide a valuable treatment option for patients at risk for sudden cardiac arrest or sudden cardiac death, especially for those who cannot get an implantable device due to cost or health issues.

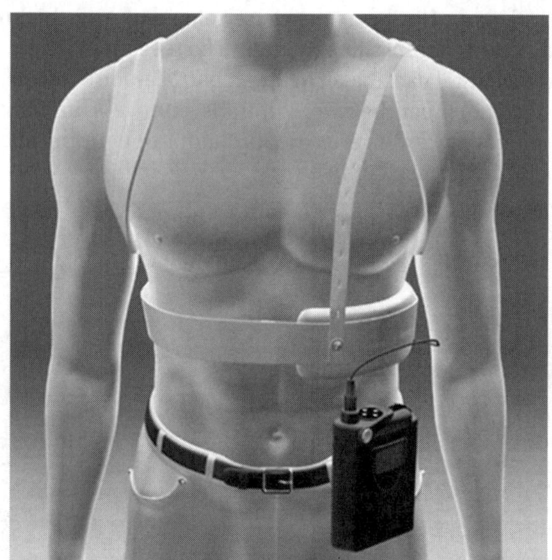

Fig. 10.11: Wearable defibrillator

How to Use an Automated External Defibrillator?

- Before using an Automated External Defibrillator (AED) on someone who you think is having Sudden Cardiac Arrest (SCA), check him/her.
- If you see a person suddenly collapse and pass out or if you find a person already unconscious, confirm that the person cannot respond.
- Shout at and shake the person to make sure he/she is not sleeping. Never shake an infant or young child. Instead, you can pinch the child to try to wake him/her up.
- Check the person's breathing and pulse. If breathing and pulse are absent or irregular, prepare to use the AED as soon as possible.
- Turn on the AED's power. The device will give you step-by-step instructions. You will hear voice prompts and see prompts on a screen. Expose the person's chest. If the person's chest is wet, dry it. AEDs have sticky pads with sensors called electrodes.
- Place one pad on the right center of the person's chest above the nipple. Place the other pad slightly below the other nipple and to the left of the ribcage.
- Remove metal necklaces and underwire bras. The metal may conduct electricity and cause burns. You can cut the center of the bra and pull it away from the skin.
- Check that the wires from the electrodes are connected to the AED. Make sure no one is touching the person and then press the AED's 'analyze' button. Stay clear while the machine checks the person's heart rhythm.
- If a shock is needed, the AED will let you know when to deliver it. Stand clear of the person and make sure others are clear before you push the AED's 'shock' button.
- Start or resume CPR until emergency medical help arrives or until the person begins to move. Report all of the information you know about what has happened.

CRASH CART

A crash cart or code cart is a set of trays/drawers/shelves on wheels used in hospitals for transportation and dispensing of emergency medication/equipment at site of medical/ surgical emergency for life support protocols (ACLS/ALS) to potentially save someone's life (Fig. 10.12).

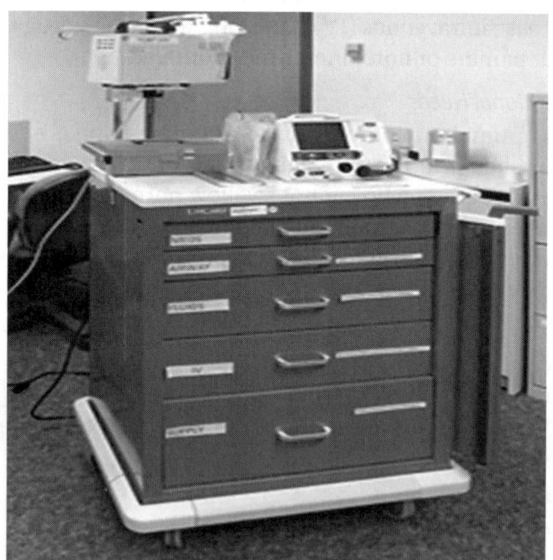

Fig. 10.12: Crash cart

The contents of a crash cart vary from hospital to hospital, but typically contain the tools and drugs needed to treat a person in or near cardiac arrest.

Hospitals typically have internal intercom codes (CODE BLUE) used for situations when someone has suffered a cardiac arrest or a similar potentially fatal condition outside of the emergency room or intensive care unit (where such conditions already happen frequently and do not require special announcements). When such codes are given, hospital staff and volunteers are expected to clear the corridors, and to direct visitors to stand aside as the crash cart and a team of physicians, pharmacists and nurses may come through at any moment. The function of a crash cart is to provide a mobile station within the hospital that contains everything needed to treat a life-threatening situation. The advantage of mobility is that it allows the treatment to come to the patient when needed.

Arrangement of Crash Cart

Top Shelf

- Defibrillator
- SpO2 probe
- Electrocardiogram (ECG) strips
- Ultrasound jelly for direct current (DC) shock
- Ambu bag for adult with mask
- Ambu bag pediatric mask. (Fig. 10.14)

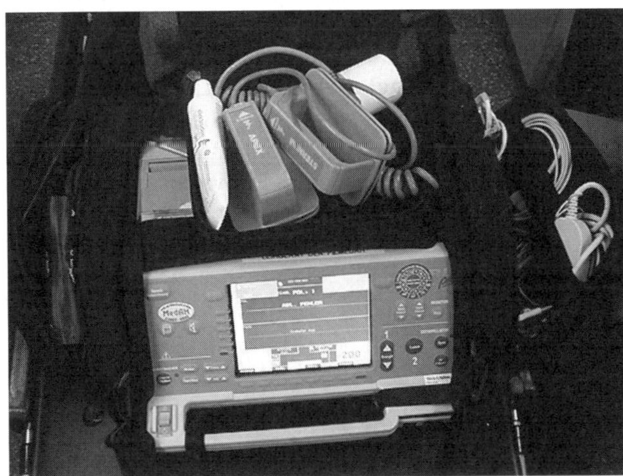

Fig. 10.13: Emergency equipment

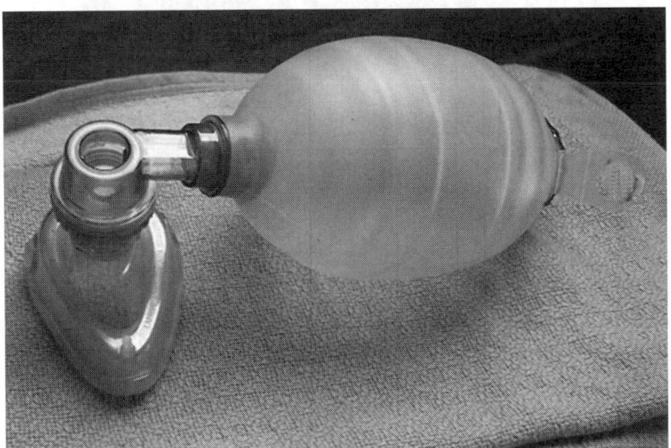

Fig. 10.14: Ambu bag pediatric mask

First Shelf (Fig. 10.15)

- Adrenaline
- Atropine sulfate
- Adenosine
- Amiodarone
- Verapamil
- Digoxin
- Dopamine
- Dobutamine
- Levophed
- Calcium gluconate
- Lasix
- Hydrocortisone
- Dilantin

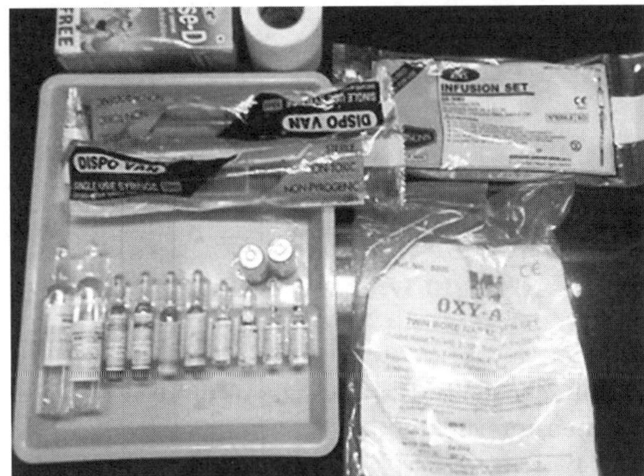

Fig. 10.15: Medication drawer tray

Second Drawer

- Dextrose 5%
- Lidocaine 1%
- Plasil
- Potassium chloride (KCl)
- Sodium bicarbonate

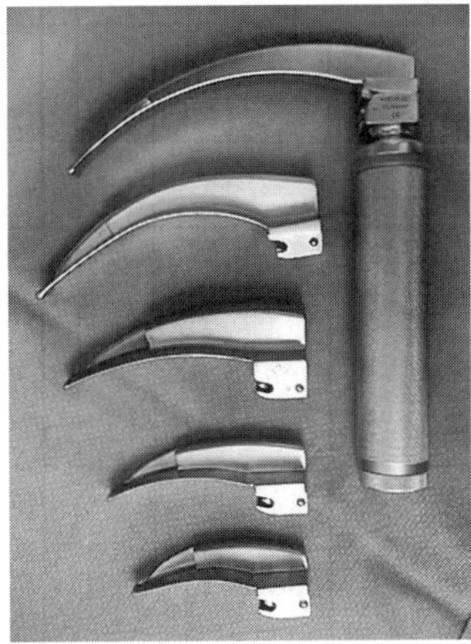

Fig. 10.16: Laryngoscope

Third Drawer

- Laryngoscope (Fig. 10.16)
- Xylocaine jelly
- Stylet
- Oropharyngeal airway
- Gauze bandage
- Plaster

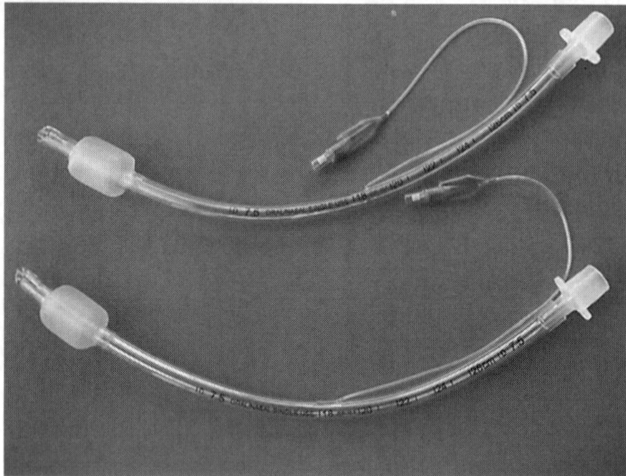

Fig. 10.17: Endotracheal tube

Fourth Drawer

- Endotracheal tube (various sizes) (Fig. 10.17)
- Tracheostomy tube
- Airway
- Suction catheters (all sizes)
- Gloves (Fig. 10.18).

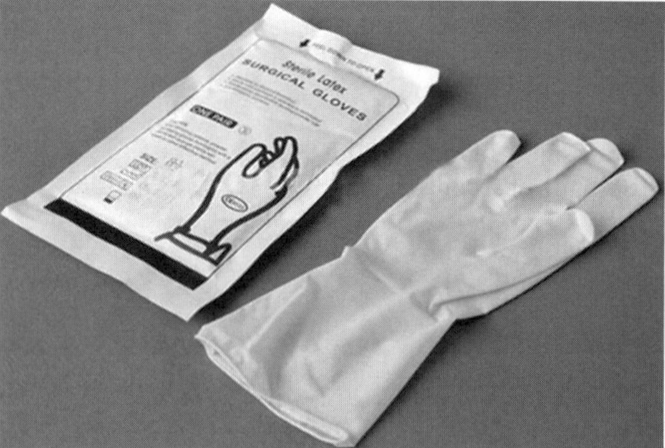

Fig. 10.18: Gloves

Nursing Responsibility

- Crash cart must be checked by head nurse/staff nurses every shift and document in checklist.
- Standardization must be maintained.
- Defibrillator will be checked by biomed department regularly or as necessary.
- Crash cart items must be checked monthly for expiry dates.
- Each unit will have crash cart placed in an easily place accessible location.

INTRAAORTIC BALLOON PUMP

The Intraaortic balloon pump (IABP) is a mechanical device that increases myocardial oxygen perfusion while at the same time increasing cardiac output. Increasing cardiac output increases coronary blood flow and therefore myocardial oxygen delivery. It consists of a cylindrical polyethylene balloon that sits in the aorta approximately 2 cm (0.79 inch) from the left subclavian artery and counterpulsates, i.e. it actively deflates in systole, increasing forward blood flow by reducing after load through a vacuum effect. It actively inflates in diastole, increasing blood flow to the coronary arteries via retrograde flow. These actions combine to decrease myocardial oxygen demand and increase myocardial oxygen supply (Fig. 10.19).

A computer controlled mechanism inflates the balloon with helium from a cylinder during diastole, usually linked to either an electrocardiogram (ECG) or a pressure transducer at the distal tip of the catheter, some IABPs, such as the datascope system 98xt, allow asynchronous counterpulsation at a set rate, though this setting is rarely used. Helium is used because its low viscosity allows it to travel quickly through the long connecting tubes, and has a lower risk than air of causing an embolism should the balloon rupture.

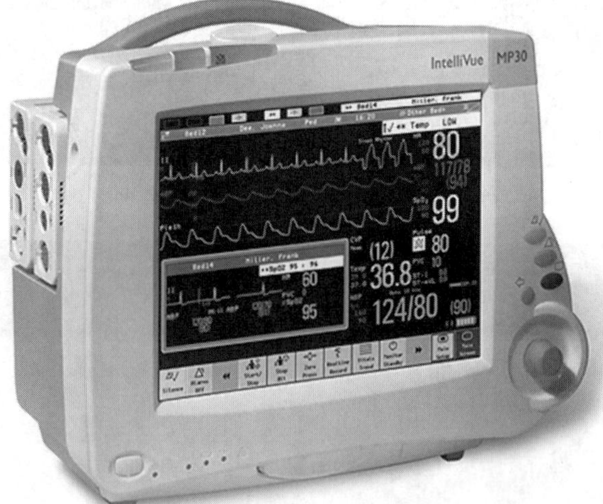

Fig. 10.19: Intraaortic balloon pump

CARDIAC MONITOR

The cardiac monitor is a device that shows the electrical and pressure waveforms of the cardiovascular system for measurement and treatment (Fig. 10.20). Parameters specific to respiratory function can also be measured. Because electrical connections are made between the cardiac monitor and the patient, it is kept at the patient's bedside.

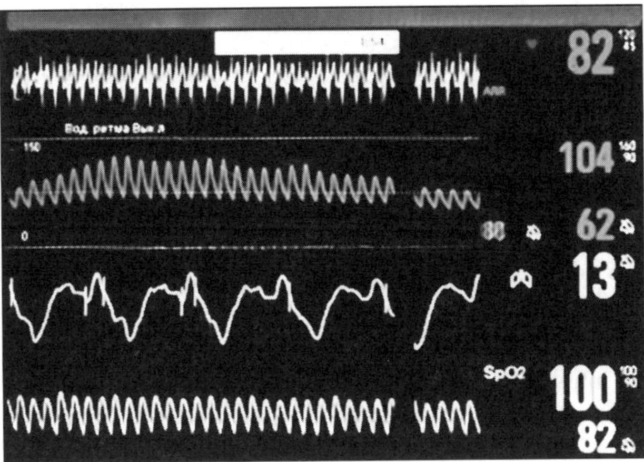

Fig. 10.20: Cardiac monitor

Purpose

The cardiac monitor continuously displays the cardiac electrocardiogram (EKG) tracing. Additional monitoring components allow cardiovascular pressures and cardiac output to be monitored and displayed as required for patient diagnosis and treatment. Oxygen saturation of the arterial blood can also be monitored continuously. Most commonly used in emergency rooms and critical care areas, bedside monitors can be interconnected to allow for continual observation of several patients from a central display. Continuous cardiovascular and pulmonary monitoring allows for prompt identification and initiation of treatment.

Description

The monitor provides a visual display of many patient parameters. It can be set to sound an alarm if any parameter changes outside of an expected range determined by the physician. Parameters to be monitored may include, but are not limited to, electrocardiogram, noninvasive blood pressure, intravascular pressures, cardiac output, arterial blood oxygen saturation,and blood temperature. Equipment required for continuous cardiac monitoring includes the cardiac monitor, cables, and disposable supplies such as electrode patches,pressure transducers, a pulmonary artery catheter (Swan-Ganz catheter), and an arterial blood saturation probe.

Preparation

As the cardiac monitor is most commonly used to monitor electrical activity of the heart, the patient can expect the following preparations. The sites selected for electrode placement on the skin is shaved and cleaned causing surface abrasion for better contact between the skin and electrode. The electrode will have a layer of gel protected by a film, which is removed prior to placing the electrode to the skin. Electrode patches will be placed near or on the right arm, right leg, left arm, left leg, and the center left side of the chest. The cable will be connected to the electrode patches for the measurement of a five-lead electrocardiogram. Additional configurations are referred to as three-lead and 12-lead electrocardiograms. If noninvasive blood pressure is being measured, a blood pressure cuff will be placed around the patient's arm or leg. The blood pressure cuff will be set to inflate manually or automatically. If manual inflation is chosen, the cuff will only inflate at the prompting of the health care provider after which a blood pressure will be displayed. During automatic operation, the blood pressure cuff will inflate at timed intervals and the display will update at the end of each measurement. The arterial blood saturation probe will be placed on the finger, toe, ear, or nasal septum of the patient providing as little discomfort as possible, while achieving a satisfactory measurement.

Aftercare

After connecting all equipment, the health care provider will observe the monitor and evaluate the quality of the tracings, while making size and position adjustments as needed. The provider will confirm that the monitor is detecting each heartbeat by taking an apical pulse and comparing the pulse to the digital display. The upper and lower alarm limits should be set according to physician orders and the alarm activated. A printout may be recorded for the medical record and labeled with patient name, room number, date, time, and interpretation of the strip. Maintenance and replacement of the disposable components may be necessary as frequently as every eight hours or as required to maintain proper operation. The arterial saturation probe can be repositioned to suit patient comfort and to obtain a tracing. All connections will be treated in a gentle manner to avoid disruption of the signal and to avoid injury to the patient.

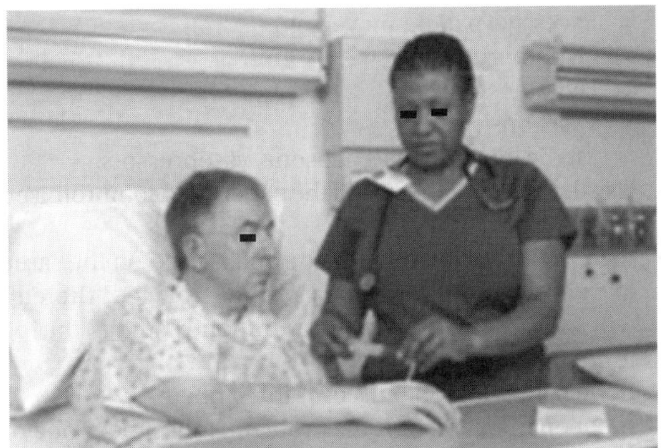

Fig. 10.21: Nurse administering IV fluid/injection

PULSE OXIMETER

Pulse oximetry is a noninvasive method for monitoring a person's O_2 saturation (Fig. 10.22). In its most common (transmissive) application mode, a sensor device is placed on a thin part of the patient's body, usually a fingertip or earlobe, or in the case of an infant, across a foot. The device passes two wavelengths of light through the body part to a photo detector. It measures the changing absorbance at each of the wavelengths allowing it to determine the absorbance due to the pulsing arterial blood alone excluding venous blood, skin, bone, muscle, fat, and nails.

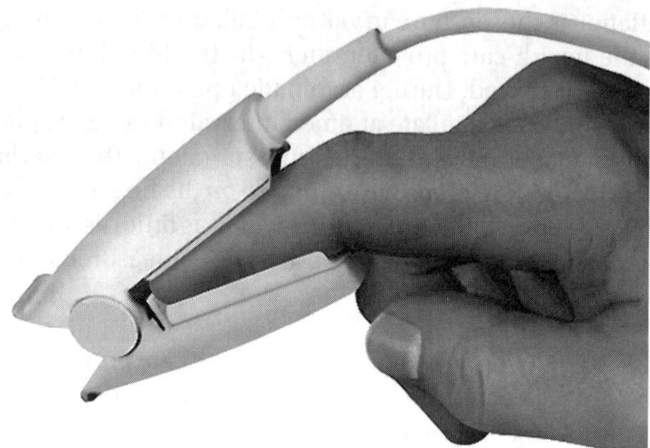

Fig. 10.22: Pulse oximeter

Nursing Interventions

Some machines have a pleth wave. A steady level even waveform ensures that the numerical reading is accurate.

- The pulse rate on the oximeter should correspond to the patient's actual pulse. If it does not, monitor the patient, check the oximeter and reposition the probe.
- Factors that interfere with accuracy include:
  - Elevated carboxyhemoglobin or methemoglobin levels
  - Lipid emulsions and dyes
  - Excessive light
  - Excessive patient movement
  - Hypothermia
  - Hypotension
  - Vasoconstriction
  - Medications such as dapsone, vasopressors.
- Use the bridge of the nose if the patient has compromised circulation in his extremities.
- If an automatic blood pressure cuff is used on the same extremity as the saturation probe is placed, the cuff will interfere with oxygen saturation readings during inflation.
- If the light is a problem, cover the probes.
- If patient movement is the problem, move the probe or select a different probe.
- Notify the physician of any significant change in the patient's condition.

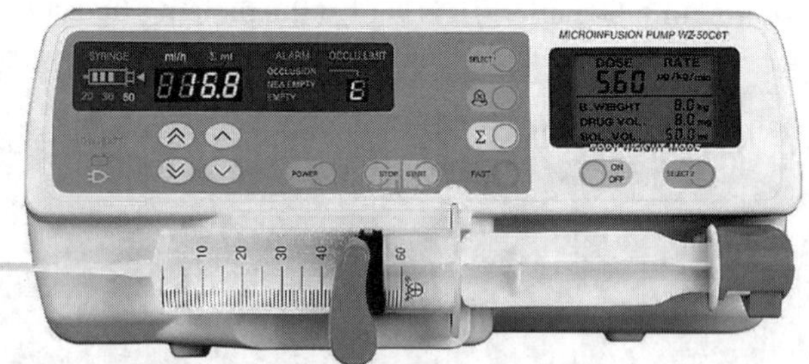

Fig. 10.23: Infusion pump

INFUSION PUMP

An infusion pump infuses fluids, medication or nutrients into a patient's circulatory system (Fig. 10.23). It is generally used intravenously, although subcutaneous, arterial and epidural infusions are occasionally used.

It can administer fluids in ways that would be impractically expensive or unreliable if performed manually by nursing staff. For example, they can administer as little as 0.1 mL per hour injections (too small for a drip), injections every minute, injections with repeated boluses requested by the patient, upto maximum number per hour (e.g. in patient-controlled analgesia), or fluids whose volumes vary by the time of day.

Because they can also produce quite high but controlled pressures, they can inject controlled amounts of fluids subcutaneously (beneath the skin) or epidurally (just within the surface of the central nervous system- a very popular local spinal anesthesia for childbirth).

Types of Infusion Pump

There are two basic classes of pumps. Large volume pumps can pump nutrient solutions large enough to feed a patient. Small volume pumps infuse hormones such as insulin or other medicines such as opiates.

1. **Large volume pumps:** They usually use some form of peristaltic pump. Classically, they use computer-controlled rollers compressing a silicone rubber tube through which the medicine flows. Another common form is a set of fingers that press on the tube in sequence.
2. **Small volume pumps:** They usually use a computer-controlled motor turning a screw that pushes the plunger on a syringe.

Nursing Interventions

- Monitor the pump and patient frequently to ensure correct operation, proper infusion rate, to detect infiltration and to observe for such complication as infection and air embolism.

- Keep the pump plugged in when possible to ensure that the battery is fully charged at all times.
- If electrical power falls, the pump will automatically switches to battery power.
- Change the tubing and cassette every 72 hours or according to facility policy.
- Reinforce the explanation of the use and purpose of the pump or controller to the patient and his family. If necessary repeat the demonstration of how the device works.

TRACHEAL TUBE

A tracheal tube is a catheter that is inserted into the trachea for the primary purpose of establishing and maintaining a patent airway and to ensure the adequate exchange of oxygen and carbon dioxide.

Many different types of tracheal tubes are available, suited for different specific applications:

- An endotracheal tube is a specific type of tracheal tube, i.e. nearly always inserted through the mouth (orotracheal) or nose (nasotracheal).
- A tracheostomy tube is another type of tracheal tube, which is 2–3 inches long (51–76 mm) curved metal or plastic tube may be inserted into a tracheostomy stoma to maintain a patent lumen.

Endotracheal Tube

Most endotracheal tubes today are constructed of polyvinyl chloride, but specialty tubes constructed of silicone rubber, latex rubber, or stainless steel are also widely available. Most tubes have an inflatable cuff to seal the trachea and bronchial tree against air leakage and aspiration of gastric contents, blood, secretions, and other fluids. Uncuffed tubes are also available, though their use is limited mostly to pediatric patients (in small children, the cricoid cartilage, the narrowest portion of the pediatric airway, often provides an adequate seal for mechanical ventilation).

Types of endotracheal tube include oral or nasal, cuffed or uncuffed, preformed, e.g. Ring, Adair, and Elwyn (RAE) tube, reinforced tubes, and double-lumen endobronchial tubes (Fig. 10.24). Tubes range in size from 2 to 10.5 mm in internal diameter (ID). The size is chosen based on the patient's body size with the smaller sizes being used for pediatric and neonatal patients.

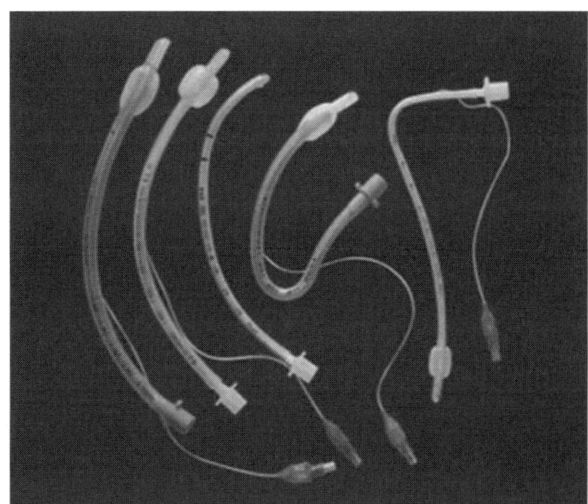

Fig. 10.24: Endotracheal tubes

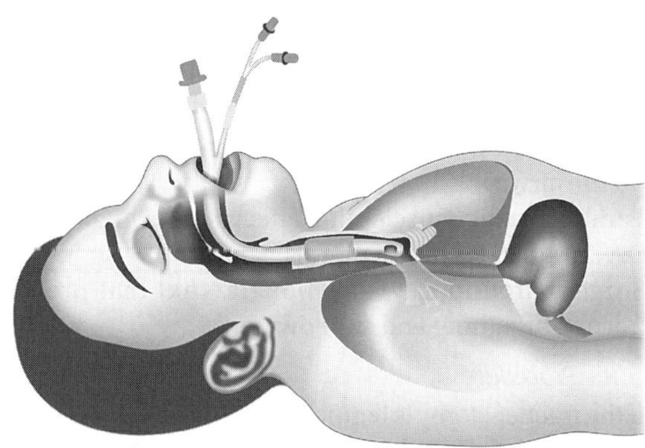

Fig. 10.25: Placement of endotracheal tube in trachea

Nursing Responsibilities for Intubated Patients

- Suctioning as needed.
- Monitoring the patient's SaO_2 by pulse oximetry as well as heart rate and blood pressure.
- Using of multiple methods to confirm correct tube placement is now a standard of care (Fig. 10.25).
- Auscultating the chest bilaterally for equal breath sounds and the abdomen for evidence of esophageal intubation.
- Endtidal CO_2 detector.
- Esophageal detection device (EDD).
- Chest X-ray.
- Keeping the head of bed elevated at 30° after intubation.

Tracheostomy Tube

A tracheostomy tube is a hollow tube with or without a cuff, i.e. that is electively inserted directly into the trachea through a surgical incision or with a wire-guided progressive dilatation technique (Figs 10.26A and B). A number of tracheostomy tubes are available for neonatal, pediatric and adult uses.

Purposes

- A large object blocking the airway.
- An inability to breathe on your own.
- An inherited abnormality of the larynx or trachea.
- Breathed in harmful material such as smoke, steam, or other toxic gases that swell and block the airway.

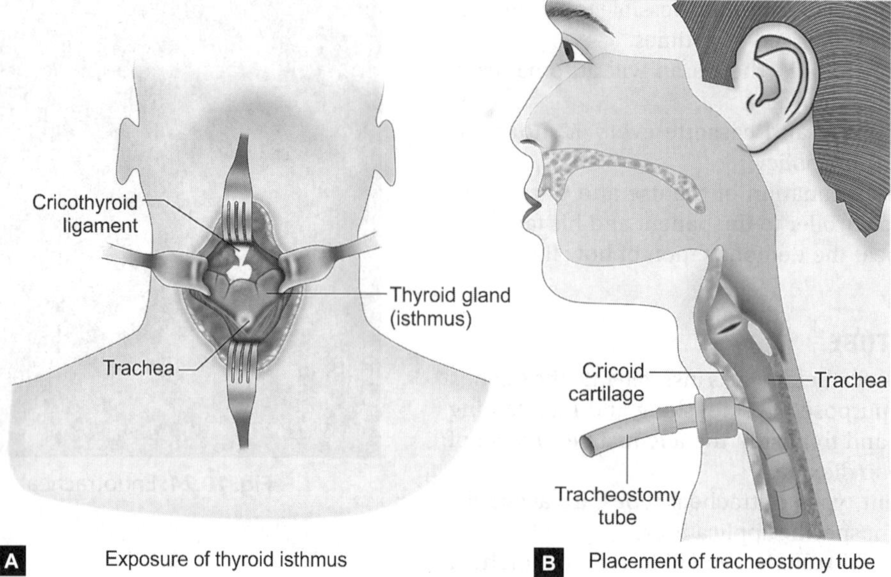

Figs 10.26A and B: Tracheostomy tube

- Cancer of the neck which can affect breathing by pressing on the airway.
- Paralysis of the muscles that affect swallowing.
- Severe neck or mouth injuries.
- Surgery around the voice box (larynx) that prevents normal breathing and swallowing.

After the Procedure

- If the tracheostomy is temporary, the tube will eventually be removed. Healing will occur quickly, leaving a minimal scar.
- Sometimes, a surgical procedure may be needed to close the site (stoma).
- Occasionally a stricture or tightening of the trachea may develop which may affect breathing.
- If the tracheostomy tube is permanent, the hole remains open.

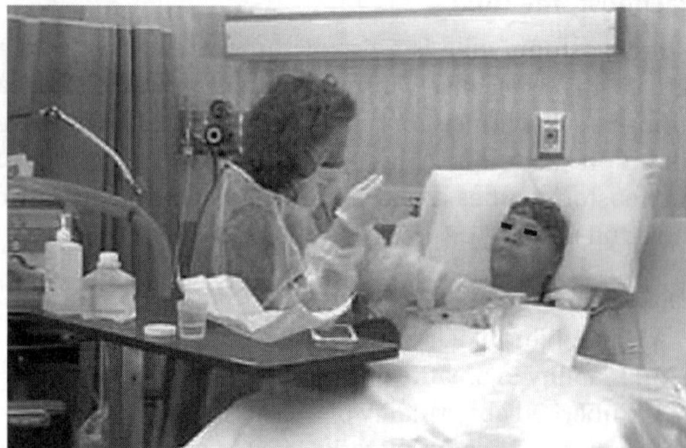

Fig. 10.27: Tracheostomy tube

NASOGASTRIC TUBE

Nasogastric intubation is a medical process involving the insertion of a plastic tube (nasogastric tube or NG tube) through the nose, past the throat, and down into the stomach (Fig. 10.28).

Purpose

A nasogastric tube is used for feeding and administering drugs and other oral agents. For drugs and for minimal quantities of liquid, a syringe is used for injection into the tube. For continuous feeding, a gravity based system is required for the feeding, the tube is often connected to an electronic pump which can control and measure the patient's intake and signal any interruption in the feeding.

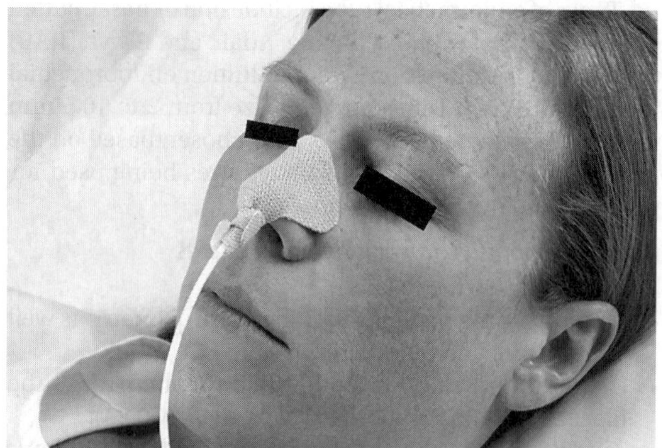

Fig. 10.28: Nasogastric tube

Contraindications

The use of nasogastric intubation is contraindicated in patients with use with base of skull fractures, severe facial fractures especially to the nose and obstructed esophagus, esophageal varices and/or obstructed airway as well as clotting disorders.

BIPAP MACHINE

Bilevel positive airway pressure (BIPAP) is a non invasive continuous positive airway pressure (CPAP) with pressure support breaths (Fig. 10.29). It is different from continuous positive airway pressure (CPAP). It delivers a preset inspiratory positive airway pressure (IPAP) during inspiration and expiratory positive airway pressure (EPAP). It can be described as a continuous positive airway pressure system with a time-cycled or flow-cycled change of the applied pressure level. Another term for bilevel positive airway pressure and the term becoming increasingly adopted by the medical community, is noninvasive positive pressure ventilation (NIPPV) or noninvasive ventilation (NIV).

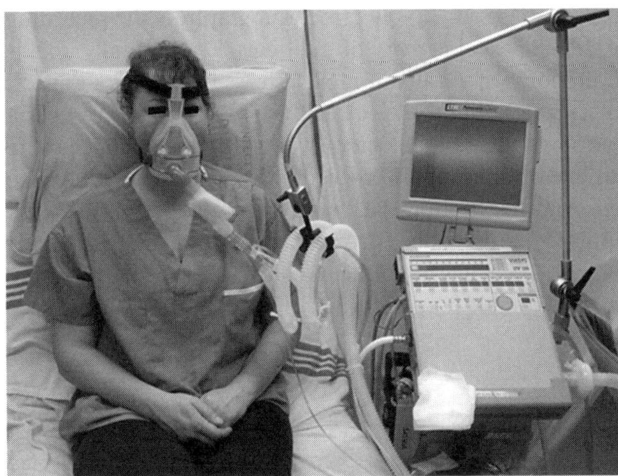

Fig. 10.29: BIPAP machine

It is used when positive airway pressure is needed with the addition of pressure support. Common situations where positive airway pressure is indicated are those where taking a breath is difficult. These include pneumonia, chronic obstructive pulmonary disease, asthma, and status asthmaticus.

SUCTION CATHETER AND MACHINE

In medicine, devices are sometimes necessary to create suction. Suction is used to clear the airway of blood, saliva, vomit, or other secretions so that a patient may breathe. Suctioning can prevent pulmonary aspiration which can lead to lung infections. In pulmonary hygiene, suction is used to remove fluids from the airways, to facilitate breathing and prevent growth of microorganisms. In surgery, suction can be used to remove blood from the area being operated on to allow surgeons to view and work on the area. It may also be used to remove blood that has built up within the skull after an intracranial hemorrhage. Suction devices may be mechanical hand pumps or battery or electrically operated mechanisms (Fig. 10.30). The plastic, rigid type of tip attached to a suction unit. Another is the plastic, nonrigid catheters sometimes called French or whistle-tip catheters.

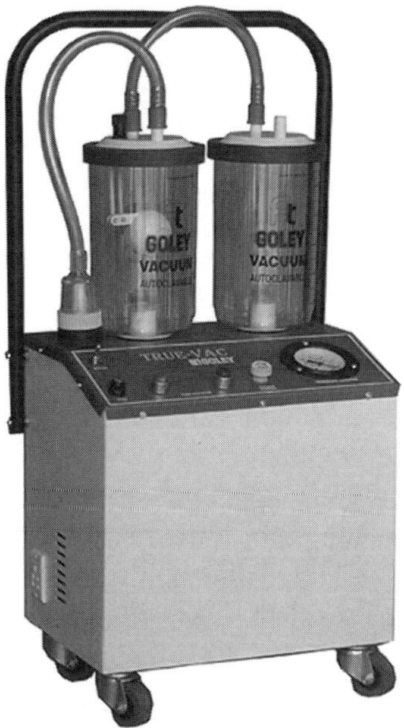

Fig. 10.30: Suction machine

CENTRAL VENOUS CATHETER

A central venous catheter ('central line', 'CVC', 'central venous line' or 'central venous access catheter') is a catheter placed into a large vein in the neck (internal jugular vein), chest (subclavian vein or axillary vein) or groin (femoral vein) (Fig. 10.31). It is used to administer medication or fluids, obtain blood tests (specifically the 'central venous oxygen saturation'), and measure central venous pressure.

Indications

Indications for the use of central lines include:

- Monitoring of the central venous pressure (CVP) in acutely ill patients to quantify fluid balance.
- Long-term intravenous antibiotics.
- Long-term parenteral nutrition especially in chronically ill patients.
- Long-term pain medications.
- Chemotherapy.

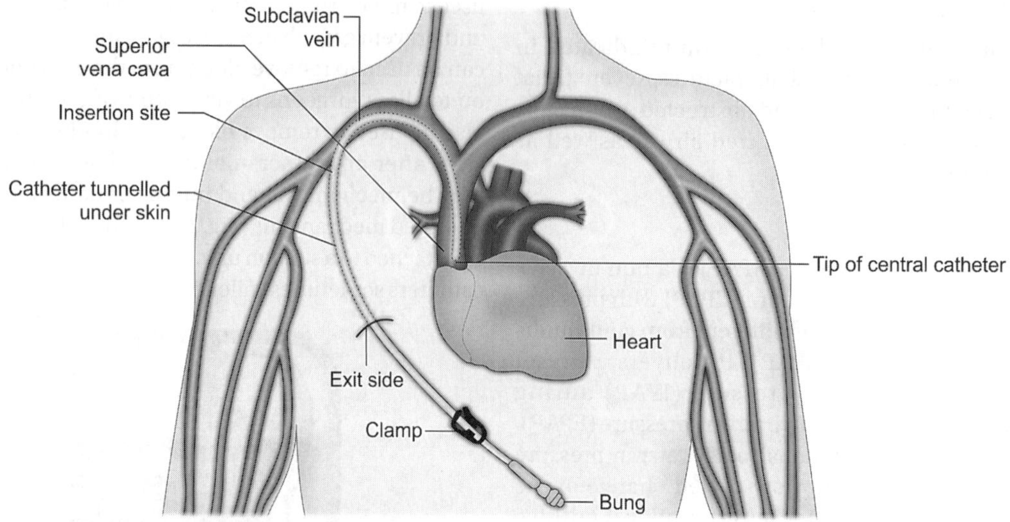

Fig. 10.31: Central venous catheter

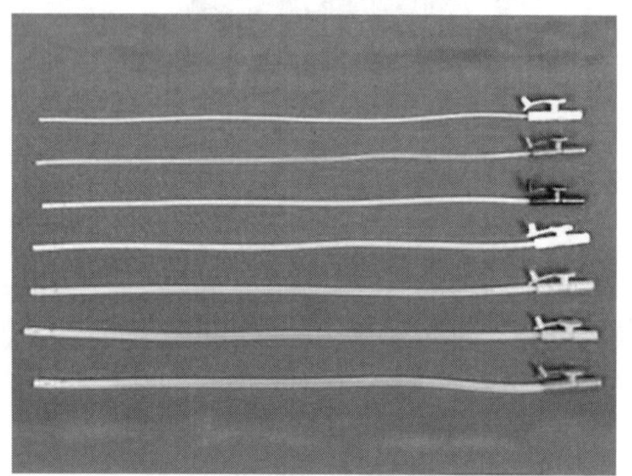

Fig. 10.32: CVP catheters

Drugs that are prone to cause phlebitis in peripheral veins (caustic) such as:

- Calcium chloride
- Chemotherapy (e.g.pentostatin, cisplatin)
- Hypertonic saline
- Potassium chloride (KCl)
- Amiodarone
- Vasopressors (e.g. epinephrine, dopamine)
- Plasmapheresis
- Peripheral blood stem cell collections
- Dialysis durgs like calcitriol, iron preparation
- Frequent blood draws
- Frequent or persistent requirement for intravenous access
- Need for intravenous therapy when peripheral venous access is impossible.
  - Blood
  - Medication
  - Rehydration.

ELECTROCARDIOGRAM (ECG) MACHINE

Electrocardiogram machine is used to measure electrocardiography (Fig. 10.33). Electrocardiography is the recording of the electrical activity of the heart. Traditionally, this is in the form of a transthoracic (across the thorax or chest) interpretation of the electrical activity of the heart over a period of time, as detected by electrodes attached to the surface of the skin and recorded or displayed by a device external to the body. The recording produced by this noninvasive procedure is termed an electrocardiogram (also ECG or EKG). It is possible to record ECGs invasively using an implantable loop recorder.

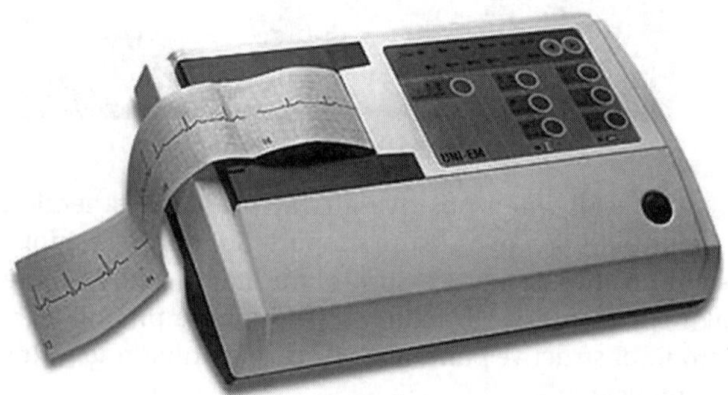

Fig. 10.33: ECG machine

An ECG is used to measure the heart's electrical conduction system. It picks up electrical impulses generated by the polarization and depolarization of cardiac tissue and translates into a waveform. The waveform is then used to measure the rate and regularity of heartbeats, as well as the size and position of the chambers, the presence of any damage to the heart, and the effects of drugs or devices used to regulate the heart such as a pacemaker.

Most ECGs are performed for diagnostic or research purposes on human hearts, but may also be performed on animals usually for diagnosis of heart abnormalities or research.

AMBU BAG

A bag valve mask, abbreviated to BVM and sometimes known by the proprietary name Ambu bag or generically as a manual resuscitator or 'self-inflating bag', is a hand-held device commonly used to provide positive pressure ventilation to patients who are not breathing or not breathing adequately. The device is a required part of resuscitation kits for trained professionals in out-of-hospital settings (such as ambulance crews) and is also frequently used in hospitals as part of standard equipment found on a crash cart, in emergency rooms or other critical care settings.

Type of Ambu Bag

Two principal types of manual resuscitator exist, one version is self-filling with air, although additional oxygen (O_2) can be added but is not necessary for the device to function. The other principal type of manual resuscitator (flow-inflation) is heavily used in non-emergent applications in the operating room to ventilate patients during anesthesia induction and recovery.

Components of Ambu Bag

Mask

Bag valve mask. Part 1 is the flexible mask to seal over the patients face, part 2 has a filter and valve to prevent backflow into the bag itself (prevents patient deprivation and bag contamination) and part 3 is the soft bag element which is squeezed to expel air to the patient. The BVM consists of a flexible air chamber (the 'bag', about the size of an American football), attached to a face mask via a shutter valve. When the face mask is properly applied and the 'bag' is squeezed, the device forces air through into the patient's lungs, when the bag is released, it self-inflates from its other end, drawing in either ambient air or a low pressure oxygen flow supplied by a regulated cylinder, while also allowing the patient's lungs to deflate to the ambient environment (not the bag) past the one way valve. (Fig. 10.34)

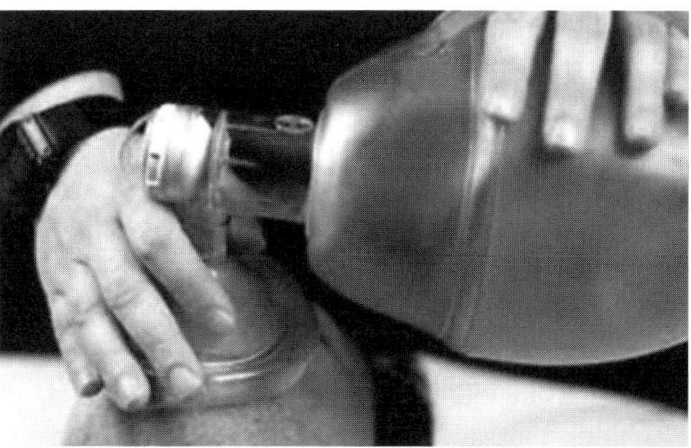

Fig. 10.34: Bag value mask

Bag and Valve

Bag and valve combinations can also be attached to an alternate airway adjunct, instead of the mask (Fig. 10.34). For example, it can be attached to an endotracheal tube or laryngeal mask airway. Small heat and moisture exchangers, or humidifying/bacterial filters can be used. A bag-valve mask can be used without being attached to an oxygen tank to provide 'room air' (21% oxygen) to the patient, however manual resuscitator devices also can be connected to a separate bag reservoir which can be filled with pure oxygen from a compressed oxygen source—this can increase the amount of oxygen delivered to the patient to nearly 100%.

Bag-valve masks come in different sizes to fit infants, children, and adults. The face mask size may be independent of the bag size, e.g. a single pediatric-sized bag might be used with different masks for multiple face sizes or a pediatric mask might be used with an adult bag for patients with small faces. Most types of the device are disposable and therefore single use, while others are designed to be cleaned and reused.

ASSIGNMENTS

I. Nursing Care Plans

II. Nursing Case Study/Presentation

III. Operation Theater Nursing

IV. Pharmacological Nursing

V. Observation Reports

VI. Procedures

I

Nursing Care Plans

Nursing Care Plan-1

Clinical Speciality________________

Identification Data:

Name:

Age:

Sex:

Hosp Regn No:

Physician:

Ward:

Bed No:

Diagnosis:

Date of admission:

Date of planning:

Physician Orders (Latest Revised):

-
-
-
-
-
-

Special Orders (Diet/Special Procedures):

-
-
-
-
-
-

Management

Medical Management:

Surgical Management (If Any):

Nursing Management

Date	Assessment	Nursing Diagnosis	Goals
			LTG: STG:

Nursing Management

Interventions	Outcome	Status of Objectives Achieved/ Reassessed

Nursing Management

Date	Assessment	Nursing Diagnosis	Goals
			LTG: STG:

Nursing Management

Interventions	Outcome	Status of Objectives Achieved/ Reassessed

Nursing Management

Date	Assessment	Nursing Diagnosis	Goals
			LTG: **STG:**

Nursing Management

Interventions	Outcome	Status of Objectives Achieved/ Reassessed

Nursing Notes

Day	Date	Vital Signs				Medication	Injection	Special Orders	IV Fluids	Nursing Remarks	Sign
		T	P	R	BP						
I											
II											
III											
IV											
V											

Nursing Care Plan-2

Clinical Speciality_______________

Identification Data:

Name:

Age:

Sex:

Hosp Regn No:

Physician:

Ward:

Bed No:

Diagnosis:

Date of admission:

Date of planning:

Physician Orders (Latest Revised):

-
-
-
-
-
-

Special Orders (Diet/Special Procedures):

-
-
-
-
-
-

Management

Medical Management:

Surgical Management (If Any):

Nursing Management

Date	Assessment	Nursing Diagnosis	Goals
			LTG: STG:

Nursing Management

Interventions	Outcome	Status of Objectives Achieved/ Reassessed

Nursing Management

Date	Assessment	Nursing Diagnosis	Goals
			LTG: **STG:**

Nursing Management

Interventions	Outcome	Status of Objectives Achieved/ Reassessed

Nursing Management

Date	Assessment	Nursing Diagnosis	Goals
			LTG: STG:

Nursing Management

Interventions	Outcome	Status of Objectives Achieved/ Reassessed

Nursing Notes

Day	Date	Vital Signs				Medication	Injection	Special Orders	IV Fluids	Nursing Remarks	Sign
		T	P	R	BP						
I											
II											
III											
IV											
V											

Nursing Care Plan-3

Clinical Speciality_______________

Identification Data:

Name:

Age:

Sex:

Hosp Regn No:

Physician:

Ward:

Bed No:

Diagnosis:

Date of admission:

Date of planning:

Physician Orders (Latest Revised):

-
-
-
-
-
-

Special Orders (Diet/Special Procedures):

-
-
-
-
-
-

Management

Medical Management:

Surgical Management (If Any):

Nursing Management

Date	Assessment	Nursing Diagnosis	Goals
			LTG: STG:

Nursing Management

Interventions	Outcome	Status of Objectives Achieved/ Reassessed

Nursing Management

Date	Assessment	Nursing Diagnosis	Goals
			LTG: **STG:**

Nursing Management

Interventions	Outcome	Status of Objectives Achieved/ Reassessed

Nursing Management

Date	Assessment	Nursing Diagnosis	Goals
			LTG: **STG:**

Nursing Management

Interventions	Outcome	Status of Objectives Achieved/ Reassessed

Nursing Notes

Day	Date	Vital Signs				Medication	Injection	Special Orders	IV Fluids	Nursing Remarks	Sign
		T	P	R	BP						
I											
II											
III											
IV											
V											

Nursing Care Plan-4

Clinical Speciality________________

Identification Data:

Name:

Age:

Sex:

Hosp Regn No:

Physician:

Ward:

Bed No:

Diagnosis:

Date of admission:

Date of planning:

Physician Orders (Latest Revised):

-
-
-
-
-
-

Special Orders (Diet/Special Procedures):

-
-
-
-
-
-

Management

Medical Management:

Surgical Management (If Any):

Nursing Management

Date	Assessment	Nursing Diagnosis	Goals
			LTG: STG:

Nursing Management

Interventions	Outcome	Status of Objectives Achieved/ Reassessed

Nursing Management

Date	Assessment	Nursing Diagnosis	Goals
			LTG: **STG:**

Nursing Management

Interventions	Outcome	Status of Objectives Achieved/ Reassessed

Nursing Management

Date	Assessment	Nursing Diagnosis	Goals
			LTG: **STG:**

Nursing Management

Interventions	Outcome	Status of Objectives Achieved/ Reassessed

Nursing Notes

Day	Date	Vital Signs				Medication	Injection	Special Orders	IV Fluids	Nursing Remarks	Sign
		T	P	R	BP						
I											
II											
III											
IV											
V											

Nursing Care Plan-5

Clinical Speciality________________

Identification Data:

Name:

Age:

Sex:

Hosp Regn No:

Physician:

Ward:

Bed No:

Diagnosis:

Date of admission:

Date of planning:

Physician Orders (Latest Revised):

•

•

•

•

•

•

Special Orders (Diet/Special Procedures):

•

•

•

•

•

•

Management

Medical Management:

Surgical Management (If Any):

Nursing Management

Date	Assessment	Nursing Diagnosis	Goals
			LTG: STG:

Nursing Management

Interventions	Outcome	Status of Objectives Achieved/ Reassessed

Nursing Management

Date	Assessment	Nursing Diagnosis	Goals
			LTG: **STG:**

Nursing Management

Interventions	Outcome	Status of Objectives Achieved/ Reassessed

Nursing Management

Date	Assessment	Nursing Diagnosis	Goals
			LTG: **STG:**

Nursing Management

Interventions	Outcome	Status of Objectives Achieved/ Reassessed

Nursing Notes

Day	Date	Vital Signs				Medication	Injection	Special Orders	IV Fluids	Nursing Remarks	Sign
		T	P	R	BP						
I											
II											
III											
IV											
V											

Nursing Care Plan-6

Clinical Speciality________________

Identification Data:

Name:

Age:

Sex:

Hosp Regn No:

Physician:

Ward:

Bed No:

Diagnosis:

Date of admission:

Date of planning:

Physician Orders (Latest Revised):

-
-
-
-
-
-

Special Orders (Diet/Special Procedures):

-
-
-
-
-
-

Management

Medical Management:

Surgical Management (If Any):

Nursing Management

Date	Assessment	Nursing Diagnosis	Goals
			LTG: **STG:**

Nursing Management

Interventions	Outcome	Status of Objectives Achieved/ Reassessed

Nursing Management

Date	Assessment	Nursing Diagnosis	Goals
			LTG: **STG:**

Nursing Management

Interventions	Outcome	Status of Objectives Achieved/ Reassessed

Nursing Management

Date	Assessment	Nursing Diagnosis	Goals
			LTG: **STG:**

Nursing Management

Interventions	Outcome	Status of Objectives Achieved/ Reassessed

Nursing Notes

Day	Date	Vital Signs				Medication	Injection	Special Orders	IV Fluids	Nursing Remarks	Sign
		T	P	R	BP						
I											
II											
III											
IV											
V											

Nursing Care Plan-7

Clinical Speciality________________

Identification Data:

Name:

Age:

Sex:

Hosp Regn No:

Physician:

Ward:

Bed No:

Diagnosis:

Date of admission:

Date of planning:

Physician Orders (Latest Revised):

-
-
-
-
-
-

Special Orders (Diet/Special Procedures):

-
-
-
-
-
-

Management

Medical Management:

Surgical Management (If Any):

Nursing Management

Date	Assessment	Nursing Diagnosis	Goals
			LTG: **STG:**

Nursing Management

Interventions	Outcome	Status of Objectives Achieved/ Reassessed

Nursing Management

Date	Assessment	Nursing Diagnosis	Goals
			LTG: STG:

Nursing Management

Interventions	Outcome	Status of Objectives Achieved/ Reassessed

Nursing Management

Date	Assessment	Nursing Diagnosis	Goals
			LTG: STG:

Nursing Management

Interventions	Outcome	Status of Objectives Achieved/ Reassessed

Nursing Notes

Day	Date	Vital Signs				Medication	Injection	Special Orders	IV Fluids	Nursing Remarks	Sign
		T	P	R	BP						
I											
II											
III											
IV											
V											

Nursing Care Plan-8

Clinical Speciality________________

Identification Data:

Name:

Age:

Sex:

Hosp Regn No:

Physician:

Ward:

Bed No:

Diagnosis:

Date of admission:

Date of planning:

Physician Orders (Latest Revised):

-
-
-
-
-
-

Special Orders (Diet/Special Procedures):

-
-
-
-
-
-

Management

Medical Management:

Surgical Management (If Any):

Nursing Management

Date	Assessment	Nursing Diagnosis	Goals
			LTG: **STG:**

Nursing Management

Interventions	Outcome	Status of Objectives Achieved/ Reassessed

Nursing Management

Date	Assessment	Nursing Diagnosis	Goals
			LTG: **STG:**

Nursing Management

Interventions	Outcome	Status of Objectives Achieved/ Reassessed

Nursing Management

Date	Assessment	Nursing Diagnosis	Goals
			LTG: **STG:**

Nursing Management

Interventions	Outcome	Status of Objectives Achieved/ Reassessed

Nursing Notes

Day	Date	Vital Signs				Medication	Injection	Special Orders	IV Fluids	Nursing Remarks	Sign
		T	P	R	BP						
I											
II											
III											
IV											
V											

Nursing Care Plan-9

Clinical Speciality_______________

Identification Data:

Name:

Age:

Sex:

Hosp Regn No:

Physician:

Ward:

Bed No:

Diagnosis:

Date of admission:

Date of planning:

Physician Orders (Latest Revised):

-
-
-
-
-
-

Special Orders (Diet/Special Procedures):

-
-
-
-
-
-

Management

Medical Management:

Surgical Management (If Any):

Nursing Management

Date	Assessment	Nursing Diagnosis	Goals
			LTG: **STG:**

Nursing Management

Interventions	Outcome	Status of Objectives Achieved/ Reassessed

Nursing Management

Date	Assessment	Nursing Diagnosis	Goals
			LTG: **STG:**

Nursing Management

Interventions	Outcome	Status of Objectives Achieved/ Reassessed

Nursing Management

Date	Assessment	Nursing Diagnosis	Goals
			LTG: **STG:**

Nursing Management

Interventions	Outcome	Status of Objectives Achieved/ Reassessed

Nursing Notes

Day	Date	Vital Signs				Medication	Injection	Special Orders	IV Fluids	Nursing Remarks	Sign
		T	P	R	BP						
I											
II											
III											
IV											
V											

Nursing Care Plan-10

Clinical Speciality_______________

Identification Data:

Name:

Age:

Sex:

Hosp Regn No:

Physician:

Ward:

Bed No:

Diagnosis:

Date of admission:

Date of planning:

Physician Orders (Latest Revised):

-
-
-
-
-
-

Special Orders (Diet/Special Procedures):

-
-
-
-
-
-

Management

Medical Management:

Surgical Management (If Any):

Nursing Management

Date	Assessment	Nursing Diagnosis	Goals
			LTG: STG:

Nursing Management

Interventions	Outcome	Status of Objectives Achieved/ Reassessed

Nursing Management

Date	Assessment	Nursing Diagnosis	Goals
			LTG: STG:

Nursing Management

Interventions	Outcome	Status of Objectives Achieved/ Reassessed

Nursing Management

Date	Assessment	Nursing Diagnosis	Goals
			LTG: **STG:**

Nursing Management

Interventions	Outcome	Status of Objectives Achieved/ Reassessed

Nursing Notes

Day	Date	Vital Signs				Medication	Injection	Special Orders	IV Fluids	Nursing Remarks	Sign
		T	P	R	BP						
I											
II											
III											
IV											
V											

Nursing Care Plan-11

Clinical Speciality_______________

Identification Data:

Name:

Age:

Sex:

Hosp Regn No:

Physician:

Ward:

Bed No:

Diagnosis:

Date of admission:

Date of planning:

Physician Orders (Latest Revised):

-
-
-
-
-
-

Special Orders (Diet/Special Procedures):

-
-
-
-
-
-

Management

Medical Management:

Surgical Management (If Any):

Nursing Management

Date	Assessment	Nursing Diagnosis	Goals
			LTG: STG:

Nursing Management

Interventions	Outcome	Status of Objectives Achieved/ Reassessed

Nursing Management

Date	Assessment	Nursing Diagnosis	Goals
			LTG: **STG:**

Nursing Management

Interventions	Outcome	Status of Objectives Achieved/ Reassessed

Nursing Management

Date	Assessment	Nursing Diagnosis	Goals
			LTG: STG:

Nursing Management

Interventions	Outcome	Status of Objectives Achieved/ Reassessed

Nursing Notes

Day	Date	Vital Signs				Medication	Injection	Special Orders	IV Fluids	Nursing Remarks	Sign
		T	P	R	BP						
I											
II											
III											
IV											
V											

Nursing Care Plan-12

Clinical Speciality________________

Identification Data:

Name:

Age:

Sex:

Hosp Regn No:

Physician:

Ward:

Bed No:

Diagnosis:

Date of admission:

Date of planning:

Physician Orders (Latest Revised):

•

•

•

•

•

•

Special Orders (Diet/Special Procedures):

•

•

•

•

•

•

Management

Medical Management:

Surgical Management (If Any):

Nursing Management

Date	Assessment	Nursing Diagnosis	Goals
			LTG: **STG:**

Nursing Management

Interventions	Outcome	Status of Objectives Achieved/ Reassessed

Nursing Management

Date	Assessment	Nursing Diagnosis	Goals
			LTG: **STG:**

Nursing Management

Interventions	Outcome	Status of Objectives Achieved/ Reassessed

Nursing Management

Date	Assessment	Nursing Diagnosis	Goals
			LTG: **STG:**

Nursing Management

Interventions	Outcome	Status of Objectives Achieved/ Reassessed

Nursing Notes

Day	Date	Vital Signs				Medication	Injection	Special Orders	IV Fluids	Nursing Remarks	Sign
		T	P	R	BP						
I											
II											
III											
IV											
V											

Nursing Care Plan-13

Clinical Speciality________________

Identification Data:

Name:

Age:

Sex:

Hosp Regn No:

Physician:

Ward:

Bed No:

Diagnosis:

Date of admission:

Date of planning:

Physician Orders (Latest Revised):

-
-
-
-
-
-

Special Orders (Diet/Special Procedures):

-
-
-
-
-
-

Management

Medical Management:

Surgical Management (If Any):

Nursing Management

Date	Assessment	Nursing Diagnosis	Goals
			LTG: STG:

Nursing Management

Interventions	Outcome	Status of Objectives Achieved/ Reassessed

Nursing Management

Date	Assessment	Nursing Diagnosis	Goals
			LTG: **STG:**

Nursing Management

Interventions	Outcome	Status of Objectives Achieved/ Reassessed

Nursing Management

Date	Assessment	Nursing Diagnosis	Goals
			LTG: **STG:**

Nursing Management

Interventions	Outcome	Status of Objectives Achieved/ Reassessed

Nursing Notes

Day	Date	Vital Signs				Medication	Injection	Special Orders	IV Fluids	Nursing Remarks	Sign
		T	P	R	BP						
I											
II											
III											
IV											
V											

Nursing Care Plan-14

Clinical Speciality________________

Identification Data:

Name:

Age:

Sex:

Hosp Regn No:

Physician:

Ward:

Bed No:

Diagnosis:

Date of admission:

Date of planning:

Physician Orders (Latest Revised):

-
-
-
-
-
-

Special Orders (Diet/Special Procedures):

-
-
-
-
-
-

Management

Medical Management:

Surgical Management (If Any):

Nursing Management

Date	Assessment	Nursing Diagnosis	Goals
			LTG: STG:

Nursing Management

Interventions	Outcome	Status of Objectives Achieved/ Reassessed

Nursing Management

Date	Assessment	Nursing Diagnosis	Goals
			LTG: **STG:**

Nursing Management

Interventions	Outcome	Status of Objectives Achieved/ Reassessed

Nursing Management

Date	Assessment	Nursing Diagnosis	Goals
			LTG: **STG:**

Nursing Management

Interventions	Outcome	Status of Objectives Achieved/ Reassessed

Nursing Notes

Day	Date	Vital Signs				Medication	Injection	Special Orders	IV Fluids	Nursing Remarks	Sign
		T	P	R	BP						
I											
II											
III											
IV											
V											

Nursing Care Plan-15

Clinical Speciality_________________

Identification Data:

Name:

Age:

Sex:

Hosp Regn No:

Physician:

Ward:

Bed No:

Diagnosis:

Date of admission:

Date of planning:

Physician Orders (Latest Revised):

-
-
-
-
-
-

Special Orders (Diet/Special Procedures):

-
-
-
-
-
-

Management

Medical Management:

Surgical Management (If Any):

Nursing Management

Date	Assessment	Nursing Diagnosis	Goals
			LTG: **STG:**

Nursing Management

Interventions	Outcome	Status of Objectives Achieved/ Reassessed

Nursing Management

Date	Assessment	Nursing Diagnosis	Goals
			LTG: **STG:**

Nursing Management

Interventions	Outcome	Status of Objectives Achieved/ Reassessed

Nursing Management

Date	Assessment	Nursing Diagnosis	Goals
			LTG: **STG:**

Nursing Management

Interventions	Outcome	Status of Objectives Achieved/ Reassessed

Nursing Notes

Day	Date	Vital Signs				Medication	Injection	Special Orders	IV Fluids	Nursing Remarks	Sign
		T	P	R	BP						
I											
II											
III											
IV											
V											

II

Nursing Case Study/ Presentation

Nursing Case Study/Presentation-1

Clinical Speciality ____________

History

i. Biographic and/or demographic details:

Name: Age: Sex: M/F

Address:

Permanent:

Present:

Hospital Registration No: ____________

Date of Admission: ____________

Ward and Unit: ____________

Bed No: ____________

Marital Status: ____________

Religion: ____________

Language: ____________

Educational qualifications: ____________

Occupation: ____________

Name of the attendant/family members: ____________

Age: ____________

Relationship with the client: ____________

Address: ____________

Diagnosis ____________

ii. Patient's reason for hospitalization:

iii. History of present illness:

Provide the details in chronological order specifying the symptoms, onset, duration, precipitating factors, relief measures adopted.

iv. Past health history:

- Past illness history

- Treatment – Surgical/Medical/Any other

- Details of previous hospitalization

- Allergies

- Menstruation

  Age at menarchy

  Regular/Irregular

  LMP

  Menopause

- Details of Immunization

- Personal habits

- Current medication being taken

- Sleeping pattern (regular/irregular/any sleep disorder)

- Any fitness/Exercise pattern

- Dietary details : Vegetarian/Nonvegetarian/Egg-vegetarian/Special diet
- Job/Work details : Any shift/Sitting or standing

v. Family history (make a family tree in the space provided and write the details):

- History of any chronic illness (DM, HTN, CAD, any other) __________
- History of any communicable disease in the family __________
- Birth/Death in family

____

vi. Environmental history:

- Drinking water supply __________
- Environmental sanitation __________
- Waste/excreta disposal __________
- Presence of flies/mosquitoes/rodents __________

vii. Psychosocial history:

- Language __________
- Details of milestones development __________
- Social support available or not __________

Physical examination (report only deviations from normal)

Diagnosis: __________

Definition

Etiology

Brief Pathophysiology

Clinical Presentation

In Literature	In Patient

Laboratory Investigations

Test	Patient Values	Normal Values

Any Advanced Test – (Report Findings)

Management

Medical Management

Drug	Dosage	Frequency	Time	Route

Surgical Management (If Any)

Operation Performed: Write Brief Details

Nursing Management

Date	Assessment	Nursing Diagnosis	Goals
			LTG: STG:

Nursing Management

Interventions	Outcome	Status of Objectives Achieved/ Reassessed

Nursing Management

Date	Assessment	Nursing Diagnosis	Goals
			LTG: **STG:**

Nursing Management

Interventions	Outcome	Status of Objectives Achieved/ Reassessed

Nursing Management

Date	Assessment	Nursing Diagnosis	Goals
			LTG: **STG:**

Nursing Management

Interventions	Outcome	Status of Objectives Achieved/ Reassessed

Nursing Notes

Day	Date	Vital Signs				Medication	Injection	Special Orders	IV Fluids	Nursing Remarks	Sign
		T	P	R	BP						
I											
II											
III											
IV											
V											

Complications

Client Education

Clinical Evaluation Remarks

Teacher's Sign

____

Nursing Case Study/Presentation-2

Clinical Speciality ____________

History

i. Biographic and/or demographic details:

Name: Age: Sex: M/F

Address:

Permanent:

Present:

Hospital Registration No: ____________

Date of Admission: ____________

Ward and Unit: ____________

Bed No: ____________

Marital Status: ____________

Religion: ____________

Language: ____________

Educational qualifications: ____________

Occupation: ____________

Name of the attendant/family members: ____________

Age: ____________

Relationship with the client: ____________

Address: ____________

Diagnosis ____________

ii. Patient's reason for hospitalization:

iii. History of present illness:

Provide the details in chronological order specifying the symptoms, onset, duration, precipitating factors, relief measures adopted.

iv. Past health history:

- Past illness history

- Treatment – Surgical/Medical/Any other

- Details of previous hospitalization

- Allergies

- Menstruation

  Age at menarchy ________

  Regular/Irregular ________

  LMP ________

  Menopause ________

- Details of Immunization

- Personal habits

- Current medication being taken

- Sleeping pattern (regular/irregular/any sleep disorder)

- Any fitness/Exercise pattern

- Dietary details : Vegetarian/Nonvegetarian/Egg-vegetarian/Special diet
- Job/Work details : Any shift/Sitting or standing

v. Family history (make a family tree in the space provided and write the details):

- History of any chronic illness (DM, HTN, CAD, any other) ____________
- History of any communicable disease in the family ____________
- Birth/Death in family

____

vi. Environmental history:

- Drinking water supply ____________
- Environmental sanitation ____________
- Waste/excreta disposal ____________
- Presence of flies/mosquitoes/rodents ____________

vii. Psychosocial history:

- Language ____________
- Details of milestones development ____________
- Social support available or not ____________

Physical examination (report only deviations from normal)

Diagnosis: ____________

Definition

Etiology

Brief Pathophysiology

Clinical Presentation

In Literature	In Patient

Laboratory Investigations

Test	Patient Values	Normal Values

Any Advanced Test – (Report Findings)

Management

Medical Management

Drug	Dosage	Frequency	Time	Route

Surgical Management (If Any)

Operation Performed: Write Brief Details

Nursing Management

Date	Assessment	Nursing Diagnosis	Goals
			LTG: STG:

Nursing Management

Interventions	Outcome	Status of Objectives Achieved/ Reassessed

Nursing Management

Date	Assessment	Nursing Diagnosis	Goals
			LTG: **STG:**

Nursing Management

Interventions	Outcome	Status of Objectives Achieved/ Reassessed

Nursing Management

Date	Assessment	Nursing Diagnosis	Goals
			LTG: **STG:**

Nursing Management

Interventions	Outcome	Status of Objectives Achieved/ Reassessed

Nursing Notes

Day	Date	Vital Signs				Medication	Injection	Special Orders	IV Fluids	Nursing Remarks	Sign
		T	P	R	BP						
I											
II											
III											
IV											
V											

Complications

Client Education

Clinical Evaluation Remarks

Teacher's Sign

____

Nursing Case Study/Presentation-3

Clinical Speciality ____________

History

i. Biographic and/or demographic details:

Name: Age: Sex: M/F

Address:

Permanent:

____

____

Present:

____

____

Hospital Registration No: ____________

Date of Admission: ____________

Ward and Unit: ____________

Bed No: ____________

Marital Status: ____________

Religion: ____________

Language: ____________

Educational qualifications: ____________

Occupation: ____________

Name of the attendant/family members: ____________

Age: ____________

Relationship with the client: ____________

Address: ____________

Diagnosis ____________

ii. Patient's reason for hospitalization:

____

____

iii. History of present illness:

Provide the details in chronological order specifying the symptoms, onset, duration, precipitating factors, relief measures adopted.

____

____

____

iv. Past health history:

____

____

- Past illness history

- Treatment – Surgical/Medical/Any other

- Details of previous hospitalization

- Allergies

- Menstruation

  Age at menarchy

  Regular/Irregular

  LMP

  Menopause

- Details of Immunization

- Personal habits

- Current medication being taken

- Sleeping pattern (regular/irregular/any sleep disorder)

- Any fitness/Exercise pattern

- Dietary details : Vegetarian/Nonvegetarian/Egg-vegetarian/Special diet
- Job/Work details : Any shift/Sitting or standing

v. Family history (make a family tree in the space provided and write the details):

- History of any chronic illness (DM, HTN, CAD, any other) ____________
- History of any communicable disease in the family ____________
- Birth/Death in family

____

vi. Environmental history:

- Drinking water supply ____________
- Environmental sanitation ____________
- Waste/excreta disposal ____________
- Presence of flies/mosquitoes/rodents ____________

vii. Psychosocial history:

- Language ____________
- Details of milestones development ____________
- Social support available or not ____________

Physical examination (report only deviations from normal)

Diagnosis: ____________

Definition

Etiology

Brief Pathophysiology

Clinical Presentation

In Literature	In Patient

Laboratory Investigations

Test	Patient Values	Normal Values

Any Advanced Test – (Report Findings)

Management

Medical Management

Drug	Dosage	Frequency	Time	Route

Surgical Management (If Any)

Operation Performed: Write Brief Details

Nursing Management

Date	Assessment	Nursing Diagnosis	Goals
			LTG: STG:

Nursing Management

Interventions	Outcome	Status of Objectives Achieved/ Reassessed

Nursing Management

Date	Assessment	Nursing Diagnosis	Goals
			LTG: **STG:**

Nursing Management

Interventions	Outcome	Status of Objectives Achieved/ Reassessed

Nursing Management

Date	Assessment	Nursing Diagnosis	Goals
			LTG: **STG:**

Nursing Management

Interventions	Outcome	Status of Objectives Achieved/ Reassessed

Nursing Notes

Day	Date	Vital Signs				Medication	Injection	Special Orders	IV Fluids	Nursing Remarks	Sign
		T	P	R	BP						
I											
II											
III											
IV											
V											

Complications

Client Education

Clinical Evaluation Remarks

Teacher's Sign

____

Nursing Case Study/Presentation-4

Clinical Speciality ____________

History

i. Biographic and/or demographic details:

Name: Age: Sex: M/F

Address:

Permanent:

Present:

Hospital Registration No: ____________

Date of Admission: ____________

Ward and Unit: ____________

Bed No: ____________

Marital Status: ____________

Religion: ____________

Language: ____________

Educational qualifications: ____________

Occupation: ____________

Name of the attendant/family members: ____________

Age: ____________

Relationship with the client: ____________

Address: ____________

Diagnosis ____________

ii. Patient's reason for hospitalization:

iii. History of present illness:

Provide the details in chronological order specifying the symptoms, onset, duration, precipitating factors, relief measures adopted.

iv. Past health history:

- Past illness history

- Treatment – Surgical/Medical/Any other

- Details of previous hospitalization

- Allergies

- Menstruation

  Age at menarchy

  Regular/Irregular

  LMP

  Menopause

- Details of Immunization

- Personal habits

- Current medication being taken

- Sleeping pattern (regular/irregular/any sleep disorder)

- Any fitness/Exercise pattern

- Dietary details : Vegetarian/Nonvegetarian/Egg-vegetarian/Special diet
- Job/Work details : Any shift/Sitting or standing

v. Family history (make a family tree in the space provided and write the details):

- History of any chronic illness (DM, HTN, CAD, any other) ______
- History of any communicable disease in the family ______
- Birth/Death in family

______

vi. Environmental history:

- Drinking water supply ______
- Environmental sanitation ______
- Waste/excreta disposal ______
- Presence of flies/mosquitoes/rodents ______

vii. Psychosocial history:

- Language ______
- Details of milestones development ______
- Social support available or not ______

Physical examination (report only deviations from normal)

Diagnosis: ______

Definition

Etiology

Brief Pathophysiology

Clinical Presentation

In Literature	In Patient

Laboratory Investigations

Test	Patient Values	Normal Values

Any Advanced Test – (Report Findings)

Management

Medical Management

Drug	Dosage	Frequency	Time	Route

Surgical Management (If Any)

Operation Performed: Write Brief Details

Nursing Management

Date	Assessment	Nursing Diagnosis	Goals
			LTG: **STG:**

Nursing Management

Interventions	Outcome	Status of Objectives Achieved/ Reassessed

Nursing Management

Date	Assessment	Nursing Diagnosis	Goals
			LTG: **STG:**

Nursing Management

Interventions	Outcome	Status of Objectives Achieved/ Reassessed

Nursing Management

Date	Assessment	Nursing Diagnosis	Goals
			LTG: STG:

Nursing Management

Interventions	Outcome	Status of Objectives Achieved/ Reassessed

Nursing Notes

Day	Date	Vital Signs				Medication	Injection	Special Orders	IV Fluids	Nursing Remarks	Sign
		T	P	R	BP						
I											
II											
III											
IV											
V											

Complications

Client Education

Clinical Evaluation Remarks

Teacher's Sign

____

Nursing Case Study/Presentation-5

Clinical Speciality ______________

History

i. Biographic and/or demographic details:

Name: Age: Sex: M/F

Address:

Permanent:

____

____

Present:

____

____

Hospital Registration No: ______________

Date of Admission: ______________

Ward and Unit: ______________

Bed No: ______________

Marital Status: ______________

Religion: ______________

Language: ______________

Educational qualifications: ______________

Occupation: ______________

Name of the attendant/family members: ______________

Age: ______________

Relationship with the client: ______________

Address: ______________

Diagnosis ______________

ii. Patient's reason for hospitalization:

____

____

iii. History of present illness:

Provide the details in chronological order specifying the symptoms, onset, duration, precipitating factors, relief measures adopted.

____

____

____

iv. Past health history:

____

____

- Past illness history

____

____

- Treatment – Surgical/Medical/Any other

____

____

- Details of previous hospitalization

____

____

- Allergies

____

____

- Menstruation

  Age at menarchy _______________

  Regular/Irregular _______________

  LMP _______________

  Menopause _______________

- Details of Immunization

____

____

- Personal habits

____

____

- Current medication being taken

____

____

____

- Sleeping pattern (regular/irregular/any sleep disorder) _______________

____

- Any fitness/Exercise pattern

____

____

- Dietary details : Vegetarian/Nonvegetarian/Egg-vegetarian/Special diet _______________
- Job/Work details : Any shift/Sitting or standing

____

____

v. Family history (make a family tree in the space provided and write the details):

- History of any chronic illness (DM, HTN, CAD, any other) __________
- History of any communicable disease in the family __________
- Birth/Death in family

____

vi. Environmental history:

- Drinking water supply __________
- Environmental sanitation __________
- Waste/excreta disposal __________
- Presence of flies/mosquitoes/rodents __________

vii. Psychosocial history:

- Language __________
- Details of milestones development __________
- Social support available or not __________

Physical examination (report only deviations from normal)

Diagnosis: __________

Definition

Etiology

Brief Pathophysiology

Clinical Presentation

In Literature	In Patient

Laboratory Investigations

Test	Patient Values	Normal Values

Any Advanced Test – (Report Findings)

Management

Medical Management

Drug	Dosage	Frequency	Time	Route

Surgical Management (If Any)

Operation Performed: Write Brief Details

Nursing Management

Date	Assessment	Nursing Diagnosis	Goals
			LTG: STG:

Nursing Management

Interventions	Outcome	Status of Objectives Achieved/ Reassessed

Nursing Management

Date	Assessment	Nursing Diagnosis	Goals
			LTG: **STG:**

Nursing Management

Interventions	Outcome	Status of Objectives Achieved/ Reassessed

Nursing Management

Date	Assessment	Nursing Diagnosis	Goals
			LTG: **STG:**

Nursing Management

Interventions	Outcome	Status of Objectives Achieved/ Reassessed

Nursing Notes

Day	Date	Vital Signs				Medication	Injection	Special Orders	IV Fluids	Nursing Remarks	Sign
		T	P	R	BP						
I											
II											
III											
IV											
V											

Complications

Client Education

Clinical Evaluation Remarks

Teacher's Sign

____

Nursing Case Study/Presentation-6

Clinical Speciality ______________

History

i. Biographic and/or demographic details:

Name: Age: Sex: M/F

Address:

Permanent:

____

____

Present:

____

____

Hospital Registration No: ______________

Date of Admission: ______________

Ward and Unit: ______________

Bed No: ______________

Marital Status: ______________

Religion: ______________

Language: ______________

Educational qualifications: ______________

Occupation: ______________

Name of the attendant/family members: ______________

Age: ______________

Relationship with the client: ______________

Address: ______________

Diagnosis ______________

ii. Patient's reason for hospitalization:

____

____

iii. History of present illness:

Provide the details in chronological order specifying the symptoms, onset, duration, precipitating factors, relief measures adopted.

____

____

____

iv. Past health history:

____

____

- Past illness history

- Treatment – Surgical/Medical/Any other

- Details of previous hospitalization

- Allergies

- Menstruation

  Age at menarchy

  Regular/Irregular

  LMP

  Menopause

- Details of Immunization

- Personal habits

- Current medication being taken

- Sleeping pattern (regular/irregular/any sleep disorder)

- Any fitness/Exercise pattern

- Dietary details : Vegetarian/Nonvegetarian/Egg-vegetarian/Special diet
- Job/Work details : Any shift/Sitting or standing

v. Family history (make a family tree in the space provided and write the details):

- History of any chronic illness (DM, HTN, CAD, any other) ______
- History of any communicable disease in the family ______
- Birth/Death in family

______

vi. Environmental history:

- Drinking water supply ______
- Environmental sanitation ______
- Waste/excreta disposal ______
- Presence of flies/mosquitoes/rodents ______

vii. Psychosocial history:

- Language ______
- Details of milestones development ______
- Social support available or not ______

Physical examination (report only deviations from normal)

Diagnosis: ______

Definition

Etiology

Brief Pathophysiology

Clinical Presentation

In Literature	In Patient

Laboratory Investigations

Test	Patient Values	Normal Values

Any Advanced Test – (Report Findings)

Management

Medical Management

Drug	Dosage	Frequency	Time	Route

Surgical Management (If Any)

Operation Performed: Write Brief Details

Nursing Management

Date	Assessment	Nursing Diagnosis	Goals
			LTG: STG:

Nursing Management

Interventions	Outcome	Status of Objectives Achieved/ Reassessed

Nursing Management

Date	Assessment	Nursing Diagnosis	Goals
			LTG: **STG:**

Nursing Management

Interventions	Outcome	Status of Objectives Achieved/ Reassessed

Nursing Management

Date	Assessment	Nursing Diagnosis	Goals
			LTG: **STG:**

Nursing Management

Interventions	Outcome	Status of Objectives Achieved/ Reassessed

Nursing Notes

Day	Date	Vital Signs				Medication	Injection	Special Orders	IV Fluids	Nursing Remarks	Sign
		T	P	R	BP						
I											
II											
III											
IV											
V											

Complications

Client Education

Clinical Evaluation Remarks

Teacher's Sign

____

Nursing Case Study/Presentation-7

Clinical Speciality ____________________

History

i. Biographic and/or demographic details:

Name: Age: Sex: M/F

Address:

Permanent:

____

____

Present:

____

____

Hospital Registration No: ____________________

Date of Admission: ____________________

Ward and Unit: ____________________

Bed No: ____________________

Marital Status: ____________________

Religion: ____________________

Language: ____________________

Educational qualifications: ____________________

Occupation: ____________________

Name of the attendant/family members: ____________________

Age: ____________________

Relationship with the client: ____________________

Address: ____

Diagnosis ____________________

ii. Patient's reason for hospitalization:

____

____

iii. History of present illness:

Provide the details in chronological order specifying the symptoms, onset, duration, precipitating factors, relief measures adopted.

____

____

____

iv. Past health history:

____

____

- Past illness history

- Treatment – Surgical/Medical/Any other

- Details of previous hospitalization

- Allergies

- Menstruation

  Age at menarchy

  Regular/Irregular

  LMP

  Menopause

- Details of Immunization

- Personal habits

- Current medication being taken

- Sleeping pattern (regular/irregular/any sleep disorder)

- Any fitness/Exercise pattern

- Dietary details : Vegetarian/Nonvegetarian/Egg-vegetarian/Special diet
- Job/Work details : Any shift/Sitting or standing

v. Family history (make a family tree in the space provided and write the details):

- History of any chronic illness (DM, HTN, CAD, any other) ____
- History of any communicable disease in the family ____
- Birth/Death in family

____

vi. Environmental history:

- Drinking water supply ____
- Environmental sanitation ____
- Waste/excreta disposal ____
- Presence of flies/mosquitoes/rodents ____

vii. Psychosocial history:

- Language ____
- Details of milestones development ____
- Social support available or not ____

Physical examination (report only deviations from normal)

Diagnosis: ____

Definition

Etiology

Brief Pathophysiology

Clinical Presentation

In Literature	In Patient

Laboratory Investigations

Test	Patient Values	Normal Values

Any Advanced Test – (Report Findings)

Management

Medical Management

Drug	Dosage	Frequency	Time	Route

Surgical Management (If Any)

Operation Performed: Write Brief Details

Nursing Management

Date	Assessment	Nursing Diagnosis	Goals
			LTG: STG:

Nursing Management

Interventions	Outcome	Status of Objectives Achieved/ Reassessed

Nursing Management

Date	Assessment	Nursing Diagnosis	Goals
			LTG: STG:

Nursing Management

Interventions	Outcome	Status of Objectives Achieved/ Reassessed

Nursing Management

Date	Assessment	Nursing Diagnosis	Goals
			LTG: STG:

Nursing Management

Interventions	Outcome	Status of Objectives Achieved/ Reassessed

Nursing Notes

Day	Date	Vital Signs				Medication	Injection	Special Orders	IV Fluids	Nursing Remarks	Sign
		T	P	R	BP						
I											
II											
III											
IV											
V											

Complications

Client Education

Clinical Evaluation Remarks

Teacher's Sign

____

Nursing Case Study/Presentation-8

Clinical Speciality ______

History

i. Biographic and/or demographic details:

Name: Age: Sex: M/F

Address:

Permanent:

Present:

Hospital Registration No: ______

Date of Admission: ______

Ward and Unit: ______

Bed No: ______

Marital Status: ______

Religion: ______

Language: ______

Educational qualifications: ______

Occupation: ______

Name of the attendant/family members: ______

Age: ______

Relationship with the client: ______

Address: ______

Diagnosis ______

ii. Patient's reason for hospitalization:

iii. History of present illness:

Provide the details in chronological order specifying the symptoms, onset, duration, precipitating factors, relief measures adopted.

iv. Past health history:

- Past illness history

- Treatment – Surgical/Medical/Any other

- Details of previous hospitalization

- Allergies

- Menstruation

  Age at menarchy

  Regular/Irregular

  LMP

  Menopause

- Details of Immunization

- Personal habits

- Current medication being taken

- Sleeping pattern (regular/irregular/any sleep disorder)

- Any fitness/Exercise pattern

- Dietary details : Vegetarian/Nonvegetarian/Egg-vegetarian/Special diet
- Job/Work details : Any shift/Sitting or standing

v. Family history (make a family tree in the space provided and write the details):

- History of any chronic illness (DM, HTN, CAD, any other) ____________
- History of any communicable disease in the family ____________
- Birth/Death in family

____

vi. Environmental history:

- Drinking water supply ____________
- Environmental sanitation ____________
- Waste/excreta disposal ____________
- Presence of flies/mosquitoes/rodents ____________

vii. Psychosocial history:

- Language ____________
- Details of milestones development ____________
- Social support available or not ____________

Physical examination (report only deviations from normal)

Diagnosis: ____________

Definition

Etiology

Brief Pathophysiology

Clinical Presentation

In Literature	In Patient

Laboratory Investigations

Test	Patient Values	Normal Values

Any Advanced Test – (Report Findings)

Management

Medical Management

Drug	Dosage	Frequency	Time	Route

Surgical Management (If Any)

Operation Performed: Write Brief Details

Nursing Management

Date	Assessment	Nursing Diagnosis	Goals
			LTG: **STG:**

Nursing Management

Interventions	Outcome	Status of Objectives Achieved/ Reassessed

Nursing Management

Date	Assessment	Nursing Diagnosis	Goals
			LTG: **STG:**

Nursing Management

Interventions	Outcome	Status of Objectives Achieved/ Reassessed

Nursing Management

Date	Assessment	Nursing Diagnosis	Goals
			LTG: STG:

Nursing Management

Interventions	Outcome	Status of Objectives Achieved/ Reassessed

Nursing Notes

Day	Date	Vital Signs				Medication	Injection	Special Orders	IV Fluids	Nursing Remarks	Sign
		T	P	R	BP						
I											
II											
III											
IV											
V											

Complications

Client Education

Clinical Evaluation Remarks

Teacher's Sign

____

Nursing Case Study/Presentation-9

Clinical Speciality ______________________

History

i. Biographic and/or demographic details:

Name: Age: Sex: M/F

Address:

Permanent:

____

____

Present:

____

____

Hospital Registration No: ______________________

Date of Admission: ______________________

Ward and Unit: ______________________

Bed No: ______________________

Marital Status: ______________________

Religion: ______________________

Language: ______________________

Educational qualifications: ______________________

Occupation: ______________________

Name of the attendant/family members: ______________________

Age: ______________________

Relationship with the client: ______________________

Address: ____

Diagnosis ______________________

ii. Patient's reason for hospitalization:

____

____

iii. History of present illness:

Provide the details in chronological order specifying the symptoms, onset, duration, precipitating factors, relief measures adopted.

____

____

____

iv. Past health history:

____

____

- Past illness history

- Treatment – Surgical/Medical/Any other

- Details of previous hospitalization

- Allergies

- Menstruation
  - Age at menarchy
  - Regular/Irregular
  - LMP
  - Menopause
- Details of Immunization

- Personal habits

- Current medication being taken

- Sleeping pattern (regular/irregular/any sleep disorder)

- Any fitness/Exercise pattern

- Dietary details : Vegetarian/Nonvegetarian/Egg-vegetarian/Special diet
- Job/Work details : Any shift/Sitting or standing

v. Family history (make a family tree in the space provided and write the details):

- History of any chronic illness (DM, HTN, CAD, any other) __________
- History of any communicable disease in the family __________
- Birth/Death in family

____

vi. Environmental history:

- Drinking water supply __________
- Environmental sanitation __________
- Waste/excreta disposal __________
- Presence of flies/mosquitoes/rodents __________

vii. Psychosocial history:

- Language __________
- Details of milestones development __________
- Social support available or not __________

Physical examination (report only deviations from normal)

Diagnosis: __________

Definition

Etiology

Brief Pathophysiology

Clinical Presentation

In Literature	In Patient

Laboratory Investigations

Test	Patient Values	Normal Values

Any Advanced Test – (Report Findings)

Management

Medical Management

Drug	Dosage	Frequency	Time	Route

Surgical Management (If Any)

Operation Performed: Write Brief Details

Nursing Management

Date	Assessment	Nursing Diagnosis	Goals
			LTG: **STG:**

Nursing Management

Interventions	Outcome	Status of Objectives Achieved/ Reassessed

Nursing Management

Date	Assessment	Nursing Diagnosis	Goals
			LTG: STG:

Nursing Management

Interventions	Outcome	Status of Objectives Achieved/ Reassessed

Nursing Management

Date	Assessment	Nursing Diagnosis	Goals
			LTG: **STG:**

Nursing Management

Interventions	Outcome	Status of Objectives Achieved/ Reassessed

Nursing Notes

Day	Date	Vital Signs				Medication	Injection	Special Orders	IV Fluids	Nursing Remarks	Sign
		T	P	R	BP						
I											
II											
III											
IV											
V											

Complications

Client Education

Clinical Evaluation Remarks

Teacher's Sign

____

Nursing Case Study/Presentation-10

Clinical Speciality ____________

History

i. Biographic and/or demographic details:

Name: Age: Sex: M/F

Address:

Permanent:

____

____

Present:

____

____

Hospital Registration No: ____________

Date of Admission: ____________

Ward and Unit: ____________

Bed No: ____________

Marital Status: ____________

Religion: ____________

Language: ____________

Educational qualifications: ____________

Occupation: ____________

Name of the attendant/family members: ____________

Age: ____________

Relationship with the client: ____________

Address: ____________

Diagnosis ____________

ii. Patient's reason for hospitalization:

____

____

iii. History of present illness:

Provide the details in chronological order specifying the symptoms, onset, duration, precipitating factors, relief measures adopted.

____

____

____

iv. Past health history:

____

____

- Past illness history

- Treatment – Surgical/Medical/Any other

- Details of previous hospitalization

- Allergies

- Menstruation

  Age at menarchy

  Regular/Irregular

  LMP

  Menopause

- Details of Immunization

- Personal habits

- Current medication being taken

- Sleeping pattern (regular/irregular/any sleep disorder)

- Any fitness/Exercise pattern

- Dietary details : Vegetarian/Nonvegetarian/Egg-vegetarian/Special diet
- Job/Work details : Any shift/Sitting or standing

v. Family history (make a family tree in the space provided and write the details):

- History of any chronic illness (DM, HTN, CAD, any other) ____________
- History of any communicable disease in the family ____________
- Birth/Death in family

____

vi. Environmental history:

- Drinking water supply ____________
- Environmental sanitation ____________
- Waste/excreta disposal ____________
- Presence of flies/mosquitoes/rodents ____________

vii. Psychosocial history:

- Language ____________
- Details of milestones development ____________
- Social support available or not ____________

Physical examination (report only deviations from normal)

Diagnosis: ____________

Definition

Etiology

Brief Pathophysiology

Clinical Presentation

In Literature	In Patient

Laboratory Investigations

Test	Patient Values	Normal Values

Any Advanced Test – (Report Findings)

Management

Medical Management

Drug	Dosage	Frequency	Time	Route

Surgical Management (If Any)

Operation Performed: Write Brief Details

Nursing Management

Date	Assessment	Nursing Diagnosis	Goals
			LTG: STG:

Nursing Management

Interventions	Outcome	Status of Objectives Achieved/ Reassessed

Nursing Management

Date	Assessment	Nursing Diagnosis	Goals
			LTG: STG:

Nursing Management

Interventions	Outcome	Status of Objectives Achieved/ Reassessed

Nursing Management

Date	Assessment	Nursing Diagnosis	Goals
			LTG: **STG:**

Nursing Management

Interventions	Outcome	Status of Objectives Achieved/ Reassessed

Nursing Notes

Day	Date	Vital Signs				Medication	Injection	Special Orders	IV Fluids	Nursing Remarks	Sign
		T	P	R	BP						
I											
II											
III											
IV											
V											

Complications

Client Education

Clinical Evaluation Remarks

Teacher's Sign

____

Nursing Case Study/Presentation-11

Clinical Speciality ______

History

i. Biographic and/or demographic details:

Name: Age: Sex: M/F

Address:

Permanent:

______

______

Present:

______

______

Hospital Registration No: ______

Date of Admission: ______

Ward and Unit: ______

Bed No: ______

Marital Status: ______

Religion: ______

Language: ______

Educational qualifications: ______

Occupation: ______

Name of the attendant/family members: ______

Age: ______

Relationship with the client: ______

Address: ______

Diagnosis ______

ii. Patient's reason for hospitalization:

______

______

iii. History of present illness:

Provide the details in chronological order specifying the symptoms, onset, duration, precipitating factors, relief measures adopted.

______

______

______

iv. Past health history:

______

______

- Past illness history

- Treatment – Surgical/Medical/Any other

- Details of previous hospitalization

- Allergies

- Menstruation

  Age at menarchy

  Regular/Irregular

  LMP

  Monopause

- Details of Immunization

- Personal habits

- Current medication being taken

- Sleeping pattern (regular/irregular/any sleep disorder)

- Any fitness/Exercise pattern

- Dietary details : Vegetarian/Nonvegetarian/Egg-vegetarian/Special diet
- Job/Work details : Any shift/Sitting or standing

v. Family history (make a family tree in the space provided and write the details):

- History of any chronic illness (DM, HTN, CAD, any other) ____________
- History of any communicable disease in the family ____________
- Birth/Death in family

____

vi. Environmental history:

- Drinking water supply ____________
- Environmental sanitation ____________
- Waste/excreta disposal ____________
- Presence of flies/mosquitoes/rodents ____________

vii. Psychosocial history:

- Language ____________
- Details of milestones development ____________
- Social support available or not ____________

Physical examination (report only deviations from normal)

Diagnosis: ____________

Definition

Etiology

Brief Pathophysiology

Clinical Presentation

In Literature	In Patient

Laboratory Investigations

Test	Patient Values	Normal Values

Any Advanced Test – (Report Findings)

Management

Medical Management

Drug	Dosage	Frequency	Time	Route

Surgical Management (If Any)

Operation Performed: Write Brief Details

Nursing Management

Date	Assessment	Nursing Diagnosis	Goals
			LTG: STG:

Nursing Management

Interventions	Outcome	Status of Objectives Achieved/ Reassessed

Nursing Management

Date	Assessment	Nursing Diagnosis	Goals
			LTG: STG:

Nursing Management

Interventions	Outcome	Status of Objectives Achieved/ Reassessed

Nursing Management

Date	Assessment	Nursing Diagnosis	Goals
			LTG: STG:

Nursing Management

Interventions	Outcome	Status of Objectives Achieved/ Reassessed

Nursing Notes

Day	Date	Vital Signs				Medication	Injection	Special Orders	IV Fluids	Nursing Remarks	Sign
		T	P	R	BP						
I											
II											
III											
IV											
V											

Complications

Client Education

Clinical Evaluation Remarks

Teacher's Sign

____

Nursing Case Study/Presentation-12

Clinical Speciality ________________

History

i. Biographic and/or demographic details:

Name: Age: Sex: M/F

Address:

Permanent:

Present:

Hospital Registration No:

Date of Admission:

Ward and Unit:

Bed No:

Marital Status:

Religion:

Language:

Educational qualifications:

Occupation:

Name of the attendant/family members:

Age:

Relationship with the client:

Address:

Diagnosis

ii. Patient's reason for hospitalization:

iii. History of present illness:

Provide the details in chronological order specifying the symptoms, onset, duration, precipitating factors, relief measures adopted.

iv. Past health history:

- Past illness history

____

____

- Treatment – Surgical/Medical/Any other

____

____

- Details of previous hospitalization

____

____

- Allergies

____

____

- Menstruation

  Age at menarchy ____________________

  Regular/Irregular ____________________

  LMP ____________________

  Menopause ____________________

- Details of Immunization

____

____

- Personal habits

____

____

- Current medication being taken

____

____

____

- Sleeping pattern (regular/irregular/any sleep disorder) ____________________

____

- Any fitness/Exercise pattern

____

____

- Dietary details : Vegetarian/Nonvegetarian/Egg-vegetarian/Special diet ____________________
- Job/Work details : Any shift/Sitting or standing

____

____

v. Family history (make a family tree in the space provided and write the details):

- History of any chronic illness (DM, HTN, CAD, any other) ____________
- History of any communicable disease in the family ____________
- Birth/Death in family

____

vi. Environmental history:

- Drinking water supply ____________
- Environmental sanitation ____________
- Waste/excreta disposal ____________
- Presence of flies/mosquitoes/rodents ____________

vii. Psychosocial history:

- Language ____________
- Details of milestones development ____________
- Social support available or not ____________

Physical examination (report only deviations from normal)

Diagnosis: ____________

Definition

Etiology

Brief Pathophysiology

Clinical Presentation

In Literature	In Patient

Laboratory Investigations

Test	Patient Values	Normal Values

Any Advanced Test – (Report Findings)

Management

Medical Management

Drug	Dosage	Frequency	Time	Route

Surgical Management (If Any)

Operation Performed: Write Brief Details

Nursing Management

Date	Assessment	Nursing Diagnosis	Goals
			LTG: **STG:**

Nursing Management

Interventions	Outcome	Status of Objectives Achieved/ Reassessed

Nursing Management

Date	Assessment	Nursing Diagnosis	Goals
			LTG: **STG:**

Nursing Management

Interventions	Outcome	Status of Objectives Achieved/ Reassessed

Nursing Management

Date	Assessment	Nursing Diagnosis	Goals
			LTG: STG:

Nursing Management

Interventions	Outcome	Status of Objectives Achieved/ Reassessed

Nursing Notes

Day	Date	Vital Signs				Medication	Injection	Special Orders	IV Fluids	Nursing Remarks	Sign
		T	P	R	BP						
I											
II											
III											
IV											
V											

Complications

Client Education

Clinical Evaluation Remarks

Teacher's Sign

____

Nursing Case Study/Presentation-13

Clinical Speciality ______________

History

i. Biographic and/or demographic details:

Name: Age: Sex: M/F

Address:

Permanent:

____

____

Present:

____

____

Hospital Registration No: ______________

Date of Admission: ______________

Ward and Unit: ______________

Bed No: ______________

Marital Status: ______________

Religion: ______________

Language: ______________

Educational qualifications: ______________

Occupation: ______________

Name of the attendant/family members: ______________

Age: ______________

Relationship with the client: ______________

Address: ______________

Diagnosis ______________

ii. Patient's reason for hospitalization:

____

____

iii. History of present illness:

Provide the details in chronological order specifying the symptoms, onset, duration, precipitating factors, relief measures adopted.

____

____

____

iv. Past health history:

____

____

- Past illness history

- Treatment – Surgical/Medical/Any other

- Details of previous hospitalization

- Allergies

- Menstruation

  Age at menarchy

  Regular/Irregular

  LMP

  Menopause

- Details of Immunization

- Personal habits

- Current medication being taken

- Sleeping pattern (regular/irregular/any sleep disorder)

- Any fitness/Exercise pattern

- Dietary details : Vegetarian/Nonvegetarian/Egg-vegetarian/Special diet
- Job/Work details : Any shift/Sitting or standing

v. Family history (make a family tree in the space provided and write the details):

- History of any chronic illness (DM, HTN, CAD, any other) ____________
- History of any communicable disease in the family ____________
- Birth/Death in family

____

vi. Environmental history:

- Drinking water supply ____________
- Environmental sanitation ____________
- Waste/excreta disposal ____________
- Presence of flies/mosquitoes/rodents ____________

vii. Psychosocial history:

- Language ____________
- Details of milestones development ____________
- Social support available or not ____________

Physical examination (report only deviations from normal)

Diagnosis: ____________

Definition

Etiology

Brief Pathophysiology

Clinical Presentation

In Literature	In Patient

Laboratory Investigations

Test	Patient Values	Normal Values

Any Advanced Test – (Report Findings)

Management

Medical Management

Drug	Dosage	Frequency	Time	Route

Surgical Management (If Any)

Operation Performed: Write Brief Details

Nursing Management

Date	Assessment	Nursing Diagnosis	Goals
			LTG: STG:

Nursing Management

Interventions	Outcome	Status of Objectives Achieved/ Reassessed

Nursing Management

Date	Assessment	Nursing Diagnosis	Goals
			LTG: STG:

Nursing Management

Interventions	Outcome	Status of Objectives Achieved/ Reassessed

Nursing Management

Date	Assessment	Nursing Diagnosis	Goals
			LTG: STG:

Nursing Management

Interventions	Outcome	Status of Objectives Achieved/ Reassessed

Nursing Notes

Day	Date	Vital Signs				Medication	Injection	Special Orders	IV Fluids	Nursing Remarks	Sign
		T	P	R	BP						
I											
II											
III											
IV											
V											

Complications

Client Education

Clinical Evaluation Remarks

Teacher's Sign

____

Nursing Case Study/Presentation-14

Clinical Speciality ____________

History

i. Biographic and/or demographic details:

Name: Age: Sex: M/F

Address:

Permanent:

____

____

Present:

____

____

Hospital Registration No: ____________

Date of Admission: ____________

Ward and Unit: ____________

Bed No: ____________

Marital Status: ____________

Religion: ____________

Language: ____________

Educational qualifications: ____________

Occupation: ____________

Name of the attendant/family members: ____________

Age: ____________

Relationship with the client: ____________

Address: ____________

Diagnosis ____________

ii. Patient's reason for hospitalization:

____

____

iii. History of present illness:

Provide the details in chronological order specifying the symptoms, onset, duration, precipitating factors, relief measures adopted.

____

____

____

iv. Past health history:

____

____

- Past illness history

- Treatment – Surgical/Medical/Any other

- Details of previous hospitalization

- Allergies

- Menstruation

  Age at menarchy

  Regular/Irregular

  LMP

  Menopause

- Details of Immunization

- Personal habits

- Current medication being taken

- Sleeping pattern (regular/irregular/any sleep disorder)

- Any fitness/Exercise pattern

- Dietary details : Vegetarian/Nonvegetarian/Egg-vegetarian/Special diet
- Job/Work details : Any shift/Sitting or standing

v. Family history (make a family tree in the space provided and write the details):

- History of any chronic illness (DM, HTN, CAD, any other) ____________
- History of any communicable disease in the family ____________
- Birth/Death in family

____

vi. Environmental history:

- Drinking water supply ____________
- Environmental sanitation ____________
- Waste/excreta disposal ____________
- Presence of flies/mosquitoes/rodents ____________

vii. Psychosocial history:

- Language ____________
- Details of milestones development ____________
- Social support available or not ____________

Physical examination (report only deviations from normal)

Diagnosis: ____________

Definition

Etiology

Brief Pathophysiology

Clinical Presentation

In Literature	In Patient

Laboratory Investigations

Test	Patient Values	Normal Values

Any Advanced Test – (Report Findings)

Management

Medical Management

Drug	Dosage	Frequency	Time	Route

Surgical Management (If Any)

Operation Performed: Write Brief Details

Nursing Management

Date	Assessment	Nursing Diagnosis	Goals
			LTG: **STG:**

Nursing Management

Interventions	Outcome	Status of Objectives Achieved/ Reassessed

Nursing Management

Date	Assessment	Nursing Diagnosis	Goals
			LTG: STG:

Nursing Management

Interventions	Outcome	Status of Objectives Achieved/ Reassessed

Nursing Management

Date	Assessment	Nursing Diagnosis	Goals
			LTG: STG:

Nursing Management

Interventions	Outcome	Status of Objectives Achieved/ Reassessed

Nursing Notes

Day	Date	Vital Signs				Medication	Injection	Special Orders	IV Fluids	Nursing Remarks	Sign
		T	P	R	BP						
I											
II											
III											
IV											
V											

Complications

Client Education

Clinical Evaluation Remarks

Teacher's Sign

____

Nursing Case Study/Presentation-15

Clinical Speciality ______

History

i. Biographic and/or demographic details:

Name: Age: Sex: M/F

Address:

Permanent:

______

______

Present:

______

______

Hospital Registration No: ______

Date of Admission: ______

Ward and Unit: ______

Bed No: ______

Marital Status: ______

Religion: ______

Language: ______

Educational qualifications: ______

Occupation: ______

Name of the attendant/family members: ______

Age: ______

Relationship with the client: ______

Address: ______

Diagnosis ______

ii. Patient's reason for hospitalization:

______

______

iii. History of present illness:

Provide the details in chronological order specifying the symptoms, onset, duration, precipitating factors, relief measures adopted.

______

______

______

iv. Past health history:

______

______

- Past illness history
- Treatment – Surgical/Medical/Any other
- Details of previous hospitalization
- Allergies
- Menstruation
  - Age at menarchy
  - Regular/Irregular
  - LMP
  - Menopause
- Details of Immunization
- Personal habits
- Current medication being taken
- Sleeping pattern (regular/irregular/any sleep disorder)
- Any fitness/Exercise pattern
- Dietary details : Vegetarian/Nonvegetarian/Egg-vegetarian/Special diet
- Job/Work details : Any shift/Sitting or standing

v. Family history (make a family tree in the space provided and write the details):

- History of any chronic illness (DM, HTN, CAD, any other) ____________
- History of any communicable disease in the family ____________
- Birth/Death in family

____

vi. Environmental history:

- Drinking water supply ____________
- Environmental sanitation ____________
- Waste/excreta disposal ____________
- Presence of flies/mosquitoes/rodents ____________

vii. Psychosocial history:

- Language ____________
- Details of milestones development ____________
- Social support available or not ____________

Physical examination (report only deviations from normal)

Diagnosis: ____________

Definition

Etiology

Brief Pathophysiology

Clinical Presentation

In Literature	In Patient

Laboratory Investigations

Test	Patient Values	Normal Values

Any Advanced Test – (Report Findings)

Management

Medical Management

Drug	Dosage	Frequency	Time	Route

Surgical Management (If Any)

Operation Performed: Write Brief Details

Nursing Management

Date	Assessment	Nursing Diagnosis	Goals
			LTG: STG:

Nursing Management

Interventions	Outcome	Status of Objectives Achieved/ Reassessed

Nursing Management

Date	Assessment	Nursing Diagnosis	Goals
			LTG: **STG:**

Nursing Management

Interventions	Outcome	Status of Objectives Achieved/ Reassessed

Nursing Management

Date	Assessment	Nursing Diagnosis	Goals
			LTG: STG:

Nursing Management

Interventions	Outcome	Status of Objectives Achieved/ Reassessed

Nursing Notes

Day	Date	Vital Signs				Medication	Injection	Special Orders	IV Fluids	Nursing Remarks	Sign
		T	P	R	BP						
I											
II											
III											
IV											
V											

Complications

Client Education

Clinical Evaluation Remarks

Teacher's Sign

____

III

Operation Theater Nursing

List down the objectives of operation theater department of your hospital.

List down the objectives of your operation theater posting.

Briefly discuss the general routine activities of operation theater.

Draw a physical layout plan of operation theater.

Write down the responsibilities of OT Head Nurse.

Discuss the responsibilities of Circulatory Nurse.

Discuss the responsibilities of Scrub Nurse.

Draw a hierarchial organization pattern of nursing personnel in OT.

Describe the role of infection control nurse in operation room.

Identify the basic equipment that you have witnessed in operation room.

List down the anesthetic agents used in various types of operative procedures (write details in pharmacology section).

Enlist the types of OT hazards. Discuss their prevention.

Identify the instruments comprising the following sets:

I. General Surgery

Basic Surgical Set	Laparotomy Set

II. Orthopedic Surgery

Basic Orthopedic Set	Knee Set	Total Hip Set

III. ENT Surgery

Basic Ear Set	Basic Nasal Set	Basic Laryngo Set

IV. Ophthalmology Set

Basic Eye Set	Basic Cataract Set

V. Gynecological Surgery

Basic Gynecological Set

VI. Plastic Surgery

General Plastic Surgery Set

VII. Urological Procedures

General Genitourinary Set (Pyeloplasty, Ureteroplasty, Prostectomy, Vasectomy Set)

Briefly discuss the methods of sterilization of instruments in OT.

Make a list of cases/surgeries in which you have acted as a Circulatory Nurse.

S. No.	Date	Patient Name	Diagnosis	Operation Performed	Surgeon	Nurse	Supervisor's Sign

Identify the cases in which you have acted as a Scrub Nurse.

S. No.	Date	Patient Name	Diagnosis	Operation Performed	Surgeon	Scrub Nurse	You have Scrubbed up Yes/No	Supervisor's Sign

Write a brief report of your OR posting with your valuable suggestions for improvization.

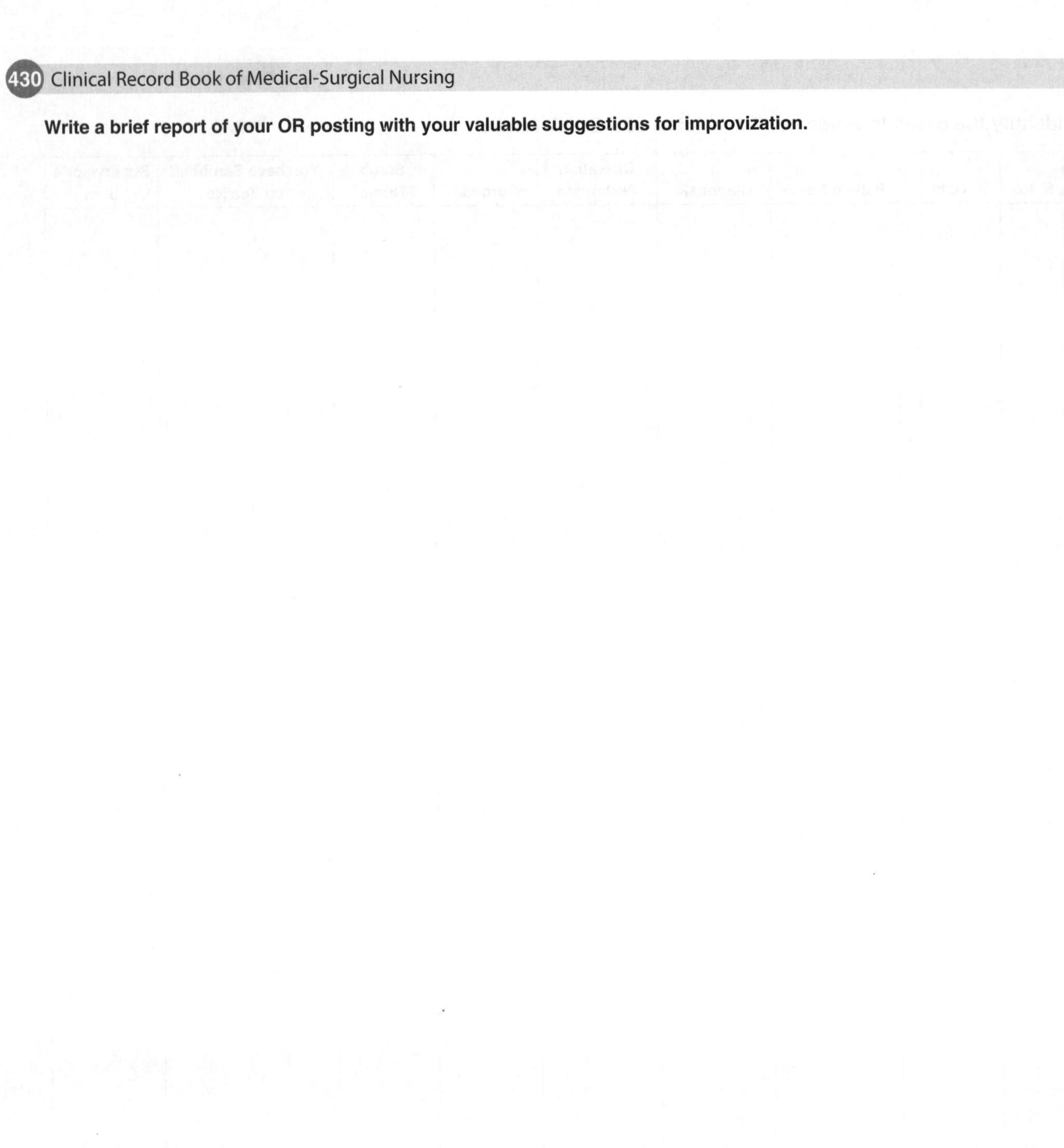

Sign of OT Teacher

____

IV

Pharmacological Nursing

Write the details of any five drugs (of each specialty) that you have learnt during your various medical-surgical clinical postings.

S. No.	Date	Drug	Clinical Specialty	Pharmacological Name	Trade Name	Dosage	Indications

Contraindications	Adverse Effects	Nursing Responsibility	Teacher's Sign

S. No.	Date	Drug	Clinical Specialty	Pharmacological Name	Trade Name	Dosage	Indications

Contraindications	Adverse Effects	Nursing Responsibility	Teacher's Sign

S. No.	Date	Drug	Clinical Specialty	Pharmacological Name	Trade Name	Dosage	Indications

Contraindications	Adverse Effects	Nursing Responsibility	Teacher's Sign

S. No.	Date	Drug	Clinical Specialty	Pharmacological Name	Trade Name	Dosage	Indications

Contraindications	Adverse Effects	Nursing Responsibility	Teacher's Sign

S. No.	Date	Drug	Clinical Specialty	Pharmacological Name	Trade Name	Dosage	Indications

Contraindications	Adverse Effects	Nursing Responsibility	Teacher's Sign

S. No.	Date	Drug	Clinical Specialty	Pharmacological Name	Trade Name	Dosage	Indications

Contraindications	Adverse Effects	Nursing Responsibility	Teacher's Sign

S. No.	Date	Drug	Clinical Specialty	Pharmacological Name	Trade Name	Dosage	Indications

Contraindications	Adverse Effects	Nursing Responsibility	Teacher's Sign

S. No.	Date	Drug	Clinical Specialty	Pharmacological Name	Trade Name	Dosage	Indications

Contraindications	Adverse Effects	Nursing Responsibility	Teacher's Sign

S. No.	Date	Drug	Clinical Specialty	Pharmacological Name	Trade Name	Dosage	Indications

Contraindications	Adverse Effects	Nursing Responsibility	Teacher's Sign

S. No.	Date	Drug	Clinical Specialty	Pharmacological Name	Trade Name	Dosage	Indications

Contraindications	Adverse Effects	Nursing Responsibility	Teacher's Sign

S. No.	Date	Drug	Clinical Specialty	Pharmacological Name	Trade Name	Dosage	Indications

Contraindications	Adverse Effects	Nursing Responsibility	Teacher's Sign

S. No.	Date	Drug	Clinical Specialty	Pharmacological Name	Trade Name	Dosage	Indications

Contraindications	Adverse Effects	Nursing Responsibility	Teacher's Sign

S. No.	Date	Drug	Clinical Specialty	Pharmacological Name	Trade Name	Dosage	Indications

Contraindications	Adverse Effects	Nursing Responsibility	Teacher's Sign

S. No.	Date	Drug	Clinical Specialty	Pharmacological Name	Trade Name	Dosage	Indications

Contraindications	Adverse Effects	Nursing Responsibility	Teacher's Sign

S. No.	Date	Drug	Clinical Specialty	Pharmacological Name	Trade Name	Dosage	Indications

Contraindications	Adverse Effects	Nursing Responsibility	Teacher's Sign

S. No.	Date	Drug	Clinical Specialty	Pharmacological Name	Trade Name	Dosage	Indications

Contraindications	Adverse Effects	Nursing Responsibility	Teacher's Sign

S. No.	Date	Drug	Clinical Specialty	Pharmacological Name	Trade Name	Dosage	Indications

Contraindications	Adverse Effects	Nursing Responsibility	Teacher's Sign

S. No.	Date	Drug	Clinical Specialty	Pharmacological Name	Trade Name	Dosage	Indications

Contraindications	Adverse Effects	Nursing Responsibility	Teacher's Sign

S. No.	Date	Drug	Clinical Specialty	Pharmacological Name	Trade Name	Dosage	Indications

Contraindications	Adverse Effects	Nursing Responsibility	Teacher's Sign

S. No.	Date	Drug	Clinical Specialty	Pharmacological Name	Trade Name	Dosage	Indications

Contraindications	Adverse Effects	Nursing Responsibility	Teacher's Sign

S. No.	Date	Drug	Clinical Specialty	Pharmacological Name	Trade Name	Dosage	Indications

Contraindications	Adverse Effects	Nursing Responsibility	Teacher's Sign

S. No.	Date	Drug	Clinical Specialty	Pharmacological Name	Trade Name	Dosage	Indications

Contraindications	Adverse Effects	Nursing Responsibility	Teacher's Sign

S. No.	Date	Drug	Clinical Specialty	Pharmacological Name	Trade Name	Dosage	Indications

Contraindications	Adverse Effects	Nursing Responsibility	Teacher's Sign

S. No.	Date	Drug	Clinical Specialty	Pharmacological Name	Trade Name	Dosage	Indications

Contraindications	Adverse Effects	Nursing Responsibility	Teacher's Sign

S. No.	Date	Drug	Clinical Specialty	Pharmacological Name	Trade Name	Dosage	Indications

Contraindications	Adverse Effects	Nursing Responsibility	Teacher's Sign

S. No.	Date	Drug	Clinical Specialty	Pharmacological Name	Trade Name	Dosage	Indications

Contraindications	Adverse Effects	Nursing Responsibility	Teacher's Sign

S. No.	Date	Drug	Clinical Specialty	Pharmacological Name	Trade Name	Dosage	Indications

Contraindications	Adverse Effects	Nursing Responsibility	Teacher's Sign

S. No.	Date	Drug	Clinical Specialty	Pharmacological Name	Trade Name	Dosage	Indications

Contraindications	Adverse Effects	Nursing Responsibility	Teacher's Sign

S. No.	Date	Drug	Clinical Specialty	Pharmacological Name	Trade Name	Dosage	Indications

Contraindications	Adverse Effects	Nursing Responsibility	Teacher's Sign

S. No.	Date	Drug	Clinical Specialty	Pharmacological Name	Trade Name	Dosage	Indications

Contraindications	Adverse Effects	Nursing Responsibility	Teacher's Sign

V

Observation Reports

Observation Report-1

Department/Area ___________

Department Objectives:

Learner's Objectives:

Physical Layout Plan of Area:

Nursing Activities:

Responsibilities of Sister In-charge:

Staffing Pattern (draw a hierarchical lineage):

Shift Duty Details:

Records and Reports:

Gadgets Available:

S. No.	Name	Purpose	Nursing Responsibilities

Policies:

1. Inventory Indent Policy

2. Waste Segregation Policy

3. Equipment Disposal Policy

Staff In-service Education:

Staff Welfare:

Observation Remarks (and any more input):

Observation Report-2

Department/Area ___________

Department Objectives:

Learner's Objectives:

Physical Layout Plan of Area:

Nursing Activities:

Responsibilities of Sister In-charge:

Staffing Pattern (draw a hierarchical lineage):

Shift Duty Details:

Records and Reports:

Gadgets Available:

S. No.	Name	Purpose	Nursing Responsibilities

Policies:

1. Inventory Indent Policy

2. Waste Segregation Policy

3. Equipment Disposal Policy

Staff In-service Education:

Staff Welfare:

Observation Remarks (and any more input):

Observation Report-3

Department/Area ____________

Department Objectives:

Learner's Objectives:

Physical Layout Plan of Area:

Nursing Activities:

Responsibilities of Sister In-charge:

Staffing Pattern (draw a hierarchical lineage):

Shift Duty Details:

Records and Reports:

Gadgets Available:

S. No.	Name	Purpose	Nursing Responsibilities

Policies:

1. Inventory Indent Policy

2. Waste Segregation Policy

3. Equipment Disposal Policy

Staff In-service Education:

Staff Welfare:

Observation Remarks (and any more input):

Observation Report-4

Department/Area ___________

Department Objectives:

Learner's Objectives:

Physical Layout Plan of Area:

Nursing Activities:

Responsibilities of Sister In-charge:

Staffing Pattern (draw a hierarchical lineage):

Shift Duty Details:

Records and Reports:

Gadgets Available:

S. No.	Name	Purpose	Nursing Responsibilities

Policies:

1. Inventory Indent Policy

2. Waste Segregation Policy

3. Equipment Disposal Policy

Staff In-service Education:

Staff Welfare:

Observation Remarks (and any more input):

Observation Report-5

Department/Area ___________

Department Objectives:

Learner's Objectives:

Physical Layout Plan of Area:

Nursing Activities:

Responsibilities of Sister In-charge:

Staffing Pattern (draw a hierarchical lineage):

Shift Duty Details:

Records and Reports:

Gadgets Available:

S. No.	Name	Purpose	Nursing Responsibilities

Policies:

1. Inventory Indent Policy

2. Waste Segregation Policy

3. Equipment Disposal Policy

Staff In-service Education:

Staff Welfare:

Observation Remarks (and any more input):

Observation Report-6

Department/Area ____________

Department Objectives:

Learner's Objectives:

Physical Layout Plan of Area:

Nursing Activities:

Responsibilities of Sister In-charge:

Staffing Pattern (draw a hierarchical lineage):

Shift Duty Details:

Records and Reports:

Gadgets Available:

S. No.	Name	Purpose	Nursing Responsibilities

Policies:

1. Inventory Indent Policy

2. Waste Segregation Policy

3. Equipment Disposal Policy

Staff In-service Education:

Staff Welfare:

Observation Remarks (and any more input):

Observation Report-7

Department/Area ___________

Department Objectives:

Learner's Objectives:

Physical Layout Plan of Area:

Nursing Activities:

Responsibilities of Sister In-charge:

Staffing Pattern (draw a hierarchical lineage):

Shift Duty Details:

Records and Reports:

Gadgets Available:

S. No.	Name	Purpose	Nursing Responsibilities

Policies:

1. Inventory Indent Policy

2. Waste Segregation Policy

3. Equipment Disposal Policy

Staff In-service Education:

Staff Welfare:

Observation Remarks (and any more input):

Observation Report-8

Department/Area ____________

Department Objectives:

Learner's Objectives:

Physical Layout Plan of Area:

Nursing Activities:

Responsibilities of Sister In-charge:

Staffing Pattern (draw a hierarchical lineage):

Shift Duty Details:

Records and Reports:

Gadgets Available:

S. No.	Name	Purpose	Nursing Responsibilities

Policies:

1. Inventory Indent Policy

2. Waste Segregation Policy

3. Equipment Disposal Policy

Staff In-service Education:

Staff Welfare:

Observation Remarks (and any more input):

Observation Report-9

Department/Area ___________

Department Objectives:

Learner's Objectives:

Physical Layout Plan of Area:

Nursing Activities:

Responsibilities of Sister In-charge:

Staffing Pattern (draw a hierarchical lineage):

Shift Duty Details:

Records and Reports:

Gadgets Available:

S. No.	Name	Purpose	Nursing Responsibilities

Policies:

1. Inventory Indent Policy

2. Waste Segregation Policy

3. Equipment Disposal Policy

Staff In-service Education:

Staff Welfare:

Observation Remarks (and any more input):

Observation Report-10

Department/Area ____________

Department Objectives:

Learner's Objectives:

Physical Layout Plan of Area:

Nursing Activities:

Responsibilities of Sister In-charge:

Staffing Pattern (draw a hierarchical lineage):

Shift Duty Details:

Records and Reports:

Gadgets Available:

S. No.	Name	Purpose	Nursing Responsibilities

Policies:

1. Inventory Indent Policy

2. Waste Segregation Policy

3. Equipment Disposal Policy

Staff In-service Education:

Staff Welfare:

Observation Remarks (and any more input):

Observation Report-11

Department/Area ___________

Department Objectives:

Learner's Objectives:

Physical Layout Plan of Area:

Nursing Activities:

Responsibilities of Sister In-charge:

Staffing Pattern (draw a hierarchical lineage):

Shift Duty Details:

Records and Reports:

Gadgets Available:

S. No.	Name	Purpose	Nursing Responsibilities

Policies:

1. Inventory Indent Policy

2. Waste Segregation Policy

3. Equipment Disposal Policy

Staff In-service Education:

Staff Welfare:

Observation Remarks (and any more input):

Observation Report-12

Department/Area ___________

Department Objectives:

Learner's Objectives:

Physical Layout Plan of Area:

Nursing Activities:

Responsibilities of Sister In-charge:

Staffing Pattern (draw a hierarchical lineage):

Shift Duty Details:

Records and Reports:

Gadgets Available:

S. No.	Name	Purpose	Nursing Responsibilities

Policies:

1. Inventory Indent Policy

2. Waste Segregation Policy

3. Equipment Disposal Policy

Staff In-service Education:

Staff Welfare:

Observation Remarks (and any more input):

Observation Report-13

Department/Area ____________

Department Objectives:

Learner's Objectives:

Physical Layout Plan of Area:

Nursing Activities:

Responsibilities of Sister In-charge:

Staffing Pattern (draw a hierarchical lineage):

Shift Duty Details:

Records and Reports:

Gadgets Available:

S. No.	Name	Purpose	Nursing Responsibilities

Policies:

1. Inventory Indent Policy

2. Waste Segregation Policy

3. Equipment Disposal Policy

Staff In-service Education:

Staff Welfare:

Observation Remarks (and any more input):

Observation Report-14

Department/Area ___________

Department Objectives:

Learner's Objectives:

Physical Layout Plan of Area:

Nursing Activities:

Responsibilities of Sister In-charge:

Staffing Pattern (draw a hierarchical lineage):

Shift Duty Details:

Records and Reports:

Gadgets Available:

S. No.	Name	Purpose	Nursing Responsibilities

Policies:

1. Inventory Indent Policy

2. Waste Segregation Policy

3. Equipment Disposal Policy

Staff In-service Education:

Staff Welfare:

Observation Remarks (and any more input):

Observation Report-15

Department/Area ____________

Department Objectives:

Learner's Objectives:

Physical Layout Plan of Area:

Nursing Activities:

Responsibilities of Sister In-charge:

Staffing Pattern (draw a hierarchical lineage):

Shift Duty Details:

Records and Reports:

Gadgets Available:

S. No.	Name	Purpose	Nursing Responsibilities

Policies:

1. Inventory Indent Policy

2. Waste Segregation Policy

3. Equipment Disposal Policy

Staff In-service Education:

Staff Welfare:

Observation Remarks (and any more input):

VI

Procedures

Procedure Record

S. No.	Name of the Procedure	Date	Teacher's Sign

I.	**MEDICAL-SURGICAL NURSING PROCEDURES (Basic and advanced)**
	• Performing medical handwashing
	• Practicing biomedical waste segregation
	• Universal precautions
	• Prevention of nosocomial infections
	• Administering total parentral nutrition
	• Administering tube feed (gastrostomy/jejunostomy)
	• Performing colostomy care
	• Performing urinary catheterization
	• Performing catheter care
	• Performing bladder irrigation
	• Removing an indwelling urinary catheter
	• Administering enema
	• Administering oxygen
	  – By mask
	  – By cannula
	  – By tent
	• Administering steam inhalation
	• Assisting a patient with incentive spirometer
	• Performing chest physiotherapy
	• Performing postural drainage
	• Performing a venipuncture
	• Administering IV infusion and care
	• Blood transfusion administration
	• Administering oral medication
	• Administering intramuscular injection
	• Administering subcutaneous injection
	• Administering intradermal injection
	• Administering medication through IV route
	• Assisting with arterial puncture
	• Performing cardiopulmonary resuscitation
	• Assisting with lumber puncture
	• Assisting with abdominal paracentesis
	• Assisting with thoracentesis
	• Assisting with endotracheal intubation
	• Assisting with bone marrow aspiration
	• Assisting with biopsy
	  – Liver
	  – Bone
	  – Kidney
	• Assessment of patient using Glasgow Coma Scale
	• Preparing a patient for advanced investigations		

S. No.	Name of the Procedure	Date	Teacher's Sign
	– MRI		
	– CT		
	– EEG		
	– ECG		
	– EMG		
	– Echocardiography		
	– Intravenous pyelography		
	– Colonoscopy		
	– Cystoscopy		
	– Rectoscopy		
	– Bronchoscopy		
	– Any other (specify)_____________		
	• Performing suctioning		
	– Oropharyngeal		
	– Trachea		
	• Performing colonic lavage/bowel wash		
	• Performing stomach wash/gastric lavage		
	• Connecting and changing intercostal drainage bottles		
	• Assisting with removal of chest drainage tubes		
	• Performing wound dressing		
	• Removal of sutures and staples		
	• Performing wound irrigation		
II.	**EMERGENCY AND ICU CARE**		
	• Care of unconscious patient		
	• Assisting defibrillation advanced cardiac life support (ACLS)		
	– Mechanical ventilators		
	– Cardiac monitor		
	• Life saving drug administration		
	• CPR		
III.	**ORTHOPEDIC NURSING**		
	• Assisting with orthopedic examination		
	• Application of splints		
	• Application of slings		
	• Applying bandages		
	• Applying binders		
	• Application of POP cast		
	• Care of patient with skin traction		
	• Care of patient with skeletal traction (pin site care)		
	• Assisting with crutch walking		
	• Assisting with walking using walker/cane		
IV.	**GYNECOLOGICAL NURSING**		
	• Preparing and assisting with gynecological examination		
	• Administering perineal care		
	• Assisting with vaginal packing		

S. No.	Name of the Procedure	Date	Teacher's Sign
	• Administering vaginal douche		
	• Administering vaginal suppository		
	• Postoperative care of gyne patient		
V.	**OPHTHALMOLOGICAL NURSING**		
	• Assisting with eye examination		
	• Eye drop instillation		
	• Eye ointment instillation		
	• Performing eye irrigation		
	• Administering eye compress (hot and cold)		
	• Administering eye care		
	• Postoperative care of patient with eye surgery		
VI.	**BURNS AND PLASTICS NURSING**		
	• Assessment/assisting with burns examination		
	• Fluid resuscitation in burn injury		
	• Topical application of medication		
	• Teaching exercises to a postburn patient		
	• Assisting with burn dressing (major)		
	• Performing minor burn bound dressing		
	• Performing wound irrigation		
	• Postoperative care of patient with plastic surgery		
VII.	**ONCOLOGY NURSING**		
	• Preparing chemotherapeutic drugs		
	• Care of patient receiving chemotherapy		
	• Care of patient undergoing radiotherapy		
	• Postoperative care of patient receiving surgical intervention		
	• Health education—patient and family		
	• Rehabilitation of cancer patient		
	• Teaching breast self examination		
	• Teaching testicular self examination		
VIII.	**OTORHINOLARYNGOLOGY NURSING**		
	• Assisting with ear examination		
	• Assisting with nasal examination		
	• Assisting with throat examination		
	• Ear drop instillation		
	• Nasal drop instillation		
	• Performing trachea suctioning		
	• Performing tracheostomy care		
	• Throat gargling		
	• Performing ear irrigation		
	• Performing nasal irrigation		
	• Postoperative care of patient with ear surgery		
	• Postoperative care of patient with nasal surgery		
	• Postoperative care of patient with laryngeal surgery		

S. No.	Name of the Procedure	Date	Teacher's Sign
IX.	**OPERATION THEATER NURSING** • Performing surgical scrub • Donning surgical attire – Gowning – Gloving – Masking – Capping • Preparing sterile field • Setting up operation theater – Operation theater carbolization – Anesthesia trolley—local, general and regional – Surgical instruments trolley – Skin preparation trolley • Preoperative preparation and assessment of patient and checklist • Intraoperative care (under anesthesia) • Immediate postoperative care of patient • Scrubbed/assisted in following surgeries – General abdominal surgery – Orthopedic surgery – ENT surgery – Gyne surgery – Eye surgery – Plastic surgery – Urology surgery • Care of instruments (post procedure) • Sterilization by – Autoclaving – Boiling – Chemical – Hot air oven • Preparation of OT articles like – Dressings – Mask/gowns/caps – Gloves – Instruments – Sutures, needles, staples – Glassware – Rubber tubing • Sending, receiving and handling of sterile supplies from CSSD • OT preparation for next day shift • Disinfection after an infected case		

S. No.	Name of the Procedure	Date	Teacher's Sign
X.	**ANY OTHER PROCEDURES (which a student has performed but is not mentioned in the section)**		

Bibliography

1. An Experienced Professor. Notes on Pathology Bacteriology, Virology and Parasitology, 9th edn, 1993, Shroff Publishers and Distributors Pvt Ltd, New Delhi.
2. Basavanthappa BT. Fundamentals of Nursing, 2nd edn, 2009, Jaypee Brothers Medical Publishers (P) Ltd, New Delhi.
3. Black JM, Hawks JH. Medical-Surgical Nursing: Clinical Management for Positive Outcomes, 7th edn, 2009, Elsevier/Saunders, St Louis.
4. Brooks SM, Waddill T. Instrumentation for the Operating Room: A Photographic Manual, 2nd edn, 2007, The CV Mosby Company.
5. Chowdhary, Sunanda S Roy. Operation Theatre Nursing, 1st edn, 2010, Kumar Publishing House, Pitampura, Delhi.
6. Heidgerken LE. Teaching and Learning in Schools of Nursing: Principles and Methods, 3rd edn, 1965, JB Lippincott, Philadelphia.
7. Jacob A et al. Clinical Nursing Procedures: The Art of Nursing Practice, 1st edn, 2010, Jaypee Brothers Medical Publishers (P) Ltd, New Delhi.
8. Kishore J. National Health Programs of India, 6th edn, 2006, Century Publications, New Delhi.
9. Linda Shields, Helen Werder. Perioperative Nursing, 2nd edn, 2010, Greenwich Medical Media (GMM), London.
10. Marilynn E Doenges, JT Burley, MF Moorhouse et al. Application of Nursing Process and Nursing Diagnosis: An Interactive Text for Diagnostic Reasoning, 3rd edn, 2000, FA Davis Company, Philadelphia.
11. Martin Hind, Paul Wicker. Principles of Perioperative Practice, 2nd edn, 2009, Churchill Livingstone. Edinburgh.
12. Moroney's Surgery for Nurses, 2nd edn, 2005, Churchill Livingstone.
13. Potter PA, Perry AG. Basic Nursing: Essentials for Practice, 5th edn, 2003, Mosby, St Louis.
14. Ruth F Craven, CH Hirnle. Fundamentals of Nursing: Human Health and Function, 4th edn, 2008, Lippincott, Philadelphia.
15. Susan S Fairchild. Perioperative Nursing Principles and Practice, 2nd edn, 1996, Little Brown and Company, Boston.
16. Taylor, Carol, Lillis et al. Fundamentals of Nursing: The Art and Science of Nursing Care, 5th edn, 2005, Lippincott Williams and Wilkins, Philadelphia.
17. Trounce John. Clinical Pharmacology for Nurses, 16th edn, 2000, Churchill Livingstone.